Occupational Therapy in Housing
Building on Firm Foundations

Occupational Therapy in Housing

Building on Firm Foundations

Edited by

SYLVIA CLUTTON Dip MCS, Dip COT, BCA,
DASEd, Certed Ed

JANI GRISBROOKE Dip COT, BA(Hons), MSc
University of Southampton

and

SUE PENGELLY Dip COT, BA(Hons), MBA, PGCE, ILTM
University of Cardiff

W
WHURR PUBLISHERS
LONDON AND PHILADELPHIA

Other Wiley Editorial Offices

John Wiley & Sons Inc., 111 River Street, Hoboken, NJ 07030, USA

Jossey-Bass, 989 Market Street, San Francisco, CA 94103-1741, USA

Wiley-VCH Verlag GmbH, Boschstr. 12, D-69469 Weinheim, Germany

John Wiley & Sons Australia Ltd, 42 McDougall Street, Milton, Queensland 4064, Australia

John Wiley & Sons (Asia) Pte Ltd, 2 Clementi Loop #02-01, Jin Xing Distripark,
Singapore 129809

John Wiley & Sons Canada Ltd, 22 Worcester Road, Etobicoke, Ontario, Canada
M9W 1L1

Wiley also publishes its books in a variety of electronic formats. Some content that
appears in print may not be available in electronic books.

A catalogue record for this book is available from the British Library

ISBN -13   978-1-86156-500-6
ISBN -10   1-86156-500-3

Printed and bound in Great Britain by TJ International Ltd, Padstow, Cornwall

This book is printed on acid-free paper responsibly manufactured from sustainable
forestry in which at least two trees are planted for each one used for paper production.

Contents

Contributors

Peter Ashlee is an experienced OT in Social Services. He has a background in the building industry and had previous architectural training. Peter is a Fieldwork Educator and is interested in the environmental effect on clients with disability, generously imparting his knowledge of relevant housing issues to student OTs.

Carla Benedict has worked in the local authority setting for 18 years. During this period, she completed further training in moving and handling and ergonomics and was Moving and Handling Specialist OT for Hampshire for three years. She is presently a senior practitioner, combining this specialist knowledge with housing adaptation work.

Sylvia Clutton, former Chair of COTSSIH and Vice Chairman of the Council of the COT, has worked in general and community health settings and managed OT services in Social Services. She works as a Consultant OT and is commissioned to provide medico-legal/judicial review/manual handling risk assessment training and housing design and redesign.

Jon Cowderoy is an experienced housing liaison officer based in the OT department. He has considerable experience of working with computer-aided design and imparting knowledge to student OTs.

Sally French works as an Associate Lecturer at the Open University and is a freelance researcher and writer. She has a particular interest in Disability Studies and has written and researched widely in this area.

Jani Grisbrooke has worked as an OT in health, local authority and education. She is currently working as a lecturer in occupational therapy for the University of Southampton and as a specialist OT in housing between Housing and Social Services Departments of Southampton City Council.

Frances Heywood is a Research Fellow at the School for Policy Studies, University of Bristol, who learnt a user-centred perspective through working for an inner-city residents' federation. She has researched widely in the field of adaptations, in partnership with occupational therapists, housing officers and disabled research colleagues.

Kathryn McNab qualified as an OT in 1985. Her first posts were hospital based, but the majority of her experience has been gained within local authority. She is currently a Team Leader with the Health and Social Care Team, a varied and demanding role including a project to incorporate smart technology into housing.

Paraig O'Brien (COTSSIH Chair) has a special interest in disability design research, completing an MA in this subject at London Guildhall University. He undertook research on assistive technologies in Oxford and more recently was seconded from the University of Ulster to assist government agencies reviewing housing adaptations services in Northern Ireland.

Sue Pengelly qualified as an OT in 1986, following which she worked in health before specialising in housing, working in both the Vale of Glamorgan and Cardiff Social Services. She is currently a Lecturer in occupational therapy at Cardiff University.

Clare Picking has worked mainly in Social Services Departments since qualifying in 1970 and as an independent practitioner for the past few years. She completed an MSc in Rehabilitation and Research and has published work on her thesis about professional roles in home adaptations in the *British Journal of Occupational Therapy*.

Samantha Pooley qualified as an OT in 2000. Following postgraduate education, her clinical practice has focused on complex moving and handling cases. She is now working as a Specialist OT for Hampshire Social Services. Ergonomic design and suitability of environments for heavier people has become a special interest for her as community 'bariatric' needs increase.

John Swain is Professor of Disability and Inclusion at the University of Northumbria. His research interests include the analysis of policy and professional practice from the viewpoints and experiences of disabled people. He has written and researched widely in this area.

Andrew Winfield has worked in local government for more than twenty years. He spent six years working in benchmarking with Welsh local government focusing on performance measurement and comparison, developing practice standards, and training and applying the principles of performance management. He has recently taken up a post with Torridge District Council in north Devon.

Preface

This book aims to provide occupational therapists with firm foundations on which to build their understanding and practice in housing work.

It grew out of the need, recognised by the College of Occupational Therapists' Specialist Section in Housing (COTSSIH), for undergraduate occupational therapists and occupational therapists newly moving into housing to have access to a text which was inspirational and drew together the various theory bases on which this eclectic aspect of the profession rested. It is part of the mission of the Specialist Section to develop this area of occupational therapy and improve outcomes for the users of our services. The editors are keen to publish a common approach to applying the principles of best practice in housing from an occupational therapy perspective in a socio-political context, where occupational therapists as designers understand the reality of the demands of the situation, the diversity of users' perspectives, building codes and statutory regulatory systems, and the regulation and inspection of their professional practice.

Designing new-build properties and redesigning properties, or parts of properties, as enabling environments in which to live and carry out meaningful occupations has been part of the core workload of occupational therapists in the UK for a very long time. The therapist generation to which the editors belong can reach back to learning from the experience of occupational therapists practising in the 1960s. This is an impressive history of practice to draw upon but has mostly been in the form of rich personal reflection on practice rather than written text.

While some areas of occupational therapy based on medical specialty can show a very well-boundaried and focused theory and evidence base, work with housing crosses a number of theory domain boundaries. The creative interaction of concepts and practices brought together by these breaches of discipline boundaries has been part of the joy of working in such a rapidly developing field.

The characteristic of practice in the field now, as in the 1960s, is that of a 'hands on' approach. Occupational therapists would wish to 'get on with the job' and find out what would work best by trying it out. These practitioners have also been curious about what related areas – ergonomics and construction disciplines, for instance – could offer in the way of ideas and support. Thus a range of theory and concepts has come into use in daily professional practice without a pressing need being felt for presenting a coherent account of them to the world. The theories and practices have been passed on from supervisor to student and shared between interested practitioners.

This book is part of the work of COTSSIH aiming to present the theory and evidence base for occupational therapy in housing in a more accessible manner for learners and all other interested parties. Having such a lively practice base, it is appropriate that a presentation of theory should grow out of that practice. The larger proportion of the authors is thus currently active as practitioner occupational therapists and others are educators and researchers in the field of occupational therapy. Alongside this, academics in social policy, disability issues and managers are represented. Although the content of this book is grounded in the experience of UK practitioners, the editors believe this situated practice which takes account of local culture, social history and legal frameworks will demonstrate principles and approaches applicable to practitioners in other countries with their own socio-political backgrounds.

The editors hope that this book conveys how challenging and satisfying such a creative endeavour as occupational therapy work in housing can be. We also hope that our service users find the outcome of those endeavours to be just as satisfying.

CHAPTER 1

The theory bases

JANI GRISBROOKE

Working with housing and people's homes, housing professionals require a different background understanding and extension of professional skills to those used to working with a healthcare team in a hospital or a community setting.

In this chapter, the theory bases which underlie what occupational therapists do with housing work, why they do it and how they do it will be examined. The sections of this chapter link to and are introductory to later chapters which cover occupational therapist practice in the field.

Theory bases identified include:

- *socio-political approaches (citizenship, rights, civil rights and social policy, control of the professions);*
- *occupational therapy approaches (problem-solving, environment as a term, Reed and Sanderson, person-environment-occupations model, Person-Environment-Occupational Performance Model, occupational science);*
- *construction and design theory bases (ergonomics, building and planning);*
- *biomedical/health theory base;*
- *two issues not in themselves theory bases (care management and evidence-based practice).*

Introduction

Working with housing means working with a phenomenon which is both universal, since most people in the world live in built accommodation, but which is culturally specific in that techniques, traditions, methods and materials for building vary across countries and ethnic groups. The experience of working with housing adaptations as an occupational therapist is also nationally specific since the ways in which adaptations for people with disabilities may be funded and the degree to which this is seen as a social or private matter vary from state to state as does underpinning legislation for regulation of building practices. This book is written from a British perspective and so, although the principles will be applicable in other states and cultures, the impact of local traditions, legislation and building practices will make some of the content specifically British.

Within this chapter, the eclectic nature of the theoretical underpinnings of occupational therapy practice with housing will be examined. Occupational therapy in housing in Britain has grown up as a praxis. Processes and ideas which had good outcomes were shared and solutions found for problems facing people living their lives in environments which provided barriers for them. A creative, problem-solving endeavour gave satisfying challenges to generations of British occupational therapists. How to manage problems has been the driver for professionals, and want of a systematic theory to account for that practice has not seemed to hold back the practitioners. Perhaps the opportunity to work in this area supported by the history of public funding of adaptations for people with disabilities has added to the growth in terms of interest and numbers of occupational therapists working in this area in Britain.

However, a need for some theory and underpinning concepts has been felt over time. Rather than systematically provide one of their own, pragmatic occupational therapists have borrowed concepts, theories and approaches from the range of other disciplines with whom they collaborate in housing work. These have become useful adjuncts to the creative process of occupational therapy. Some of the major borrowings are considered in this chapter alongside the unfinished task of theorising environmental and housing work from an occupational therapy perspective. This is a critical time for occupational therapy theory in the housing domain as the drive to ground practice in evidence directs professions to systematise their knowledge and skill bases, and so this is also a good time to review the theory bases from which occupational therapists operate.

Range of theory bases

For people who use the services of an occupational therapist (OT) within a housing context, the OT will access:

- theory bases underpinning and forming the service within which the OT is situated (*socio-political approaches*);
- a theory and skill base of occupational therapy appropriate to the service user's needs (*OT approaches*);
- theory bases of design and construction (*ergonomics and building/designing/planning approaches*);

- a theory base about impairment and medical pathology if this is relevant to the service user's situation (*biomedical science*);
- factors which affect practice but which are not in themselves theory bases (*care management and evidence-based practice*).

Socio-political approaches

The themes chosen to introduce some socio-political approaches – citizenship and rights, people and professionals – are currently contested issues with direct impact on professionals, services and people who access those services.

Citizenship in Britain

Our understanding of who our service is for as occupational therapists, what it is for and how it is delivered can be shaped subtly by the situation in which we are working. For housing work within a local authority context (which is where the majority but not all of it happens), occupational therapists are currently delivering a service to citizens who have a right to that service (DoH, 1998). Occupational therapists therefore need to appreciate the current debates around the issue of citizenship in order to frame services appropriately through understanding what it means to be a citizen.

Citizenship is an identity which has been increasingly discussed politically and in the media since the 1990s, but citizenship can mean different things in different contexts. The idea of 'good citizenship' embodied in the Neighbourhood Watch, a government-sponsored scheme by which people volunteer to look out for untoward occurrences in their own street, may not necessarily be the same citizenship envisaged in housing policy such as social landlordship with respect to housing associations, which are organisations designed to provide affordable housing for rent. Two ways of being a good citizen are illustrated in these examples. The first can be interpreted as making sure that fellow citizens' property-owning and public service rights are respected. Here individual citizens 'own' property and public service rights and a fellow citizen's duty is to support these rights. The second can be interpreted as recognising that not all people in society have the same opportunities and possibilities but, as fellow citizens, still have rights to a reasonable standard of living. Here the citizen has a duty within society as a whole to support its weaker members. So citizenship is a term which can be applied with some flexibility of meaning.

Heater (1990) suggests that citizenship is a dual form of identity. At one level 'A citizen is someone who has political freedom and responsibility'

(p. 183). She has grown into this freedom socially through participation in society and education. At another level, citizenship may be the common overlay to diverse cultural identities so that the identity of 'Britishness' covers people from Newcastle and St Ives, lorry drivers and theatre designers, humanists and Muslims, people of Norman descent and people of Afro-Caribbean descent. On the other hand, citizenship of Manchester may be of much more personal significance than citizenship of Britain. These citizenships may even be in conflict if local and national policies (e.g. employment, housing, education) are not in harmony. Currently, with devolution of powers from Westminster to the Scottish Parliament and Welsh Assembly (the situation in Northern Ireland is a little more complex), we are also struggling with Welsh, Scottish, Irish and English citizen identities over and against Britishness. Clearly, citizenship is a shifting concept, a shifting identity. However, as occupational therapists we have to struggle with the concept and the identities because on them depends whom we serve and how.

Rights

Citizens have rights and obligations to each other and to the state from which they derive that citizenship. Rights come in a variety of categories: positive (the right to something), negative (the right not to have something inflicted on you), human (the right not to be tortured or suffer inhuman treatment), political (the right to vote), civil (the right to freedom from discrimination on grounds of gender) and finally a contested category of social and economic rights (to education and a basic wage) (Plant, 1991).

Rights shift within a cultural and political context and between states. They are upholdable in law and many have reciprocal obligations attached. For instance, the right to education for all children in this country comes under the Education Acts (1944, 1981, 1993, 1996). The obligation on the parents is to ensure that their children attend that educational provision.

If rights are not upholdable in law, it is debatable whether they exist or are simply custom and practice. Thus it is worth clarifying which of your client's rights *are* rights and which are local practice. For instance, the mandatory Disabled Facilities Grant, which is the statutory provision available to people with disabilities to make alterations to the structure of the home so that essential facilities are available to them, is upholdable in housing law. However, if facilities and equipment are provided alongside this, they may be assessed by criteria agreed locally and so provision of these will be a softer right and will vary from local authority to local authority. Even these softer rights may have some basis in legal guidelines established through case law (i.e. the body of legal decisions made on particular cases and which are applied to subsequent cases which have similar principles involved). Such guidelines could offer support for a challenge in the courts to local practice. These points illustrate why an occupational therapist needs an underpinning knowledge of the complex areas of housing and community care law (Mandelstam, 1998). Also bear in mind that law, and particularly its interpretation in cases, changes over time. For instance, we are currently witnessing the impact of the Human Rights Act 1998 on a variety of areas of practice, and so a practitioner's knowledge in this area will need updating.

Civil rights

The right for all citizens to have an equal opportunity to participate in society, in political activity, education and work, has been upheld in the various anti-discrimination laws, most recently disability anti-discrimination legislation in the Disability Discrimination Act 1995.

The passing of this Act was an interesting illustration of the conflict between a rights-based view of disability affecting all areas of life and the tendency of our central political administration to deal with issues in a fragmented manner within established bureaucratic departments. Departments responsible for health care, education and housing all have a responsibility for aspects of the lives of people with disability. It was also an illustration of vested economic interests, such as the construction industry, being drawn into the political process and of cross-party support for a particular issue raised by the various organisations which make up the disability movement (Goldsmith, 1997).

The position of the disability movement is based in the establishment of the Social Model of Disability as opposed to the Medical Model (Oliver, 1999). Within this model, disability is not the tragic consequence of impairment to the individual but is a problem of a society which creates barriers to the individual's participation in society. Thus it is not the problem of the individual that wheelchair access is denied but the problem of a society which allows the construction of buildings which shut people out. Goldsmith (1997) goes further and identifies a form of architectural discrimination by which the design of buildings makes them difficult to use not only for people with specific impairments but also, for example, for women with children.

The problem of the fragmentation of responsibility for disability rights between a range of statutes and government departments was compounded by the problem of the difference previously referred to between rights which are available in law and rights which are accessible. So, for instance, you will only claim a right if you are aware of it (i.e. is you are aware that you have an entitlement to service or facility provision under particular legislation) and if the local system for advice and funding is in place by which you can put it into operation.

The Disability Discrimination Act 1995 did not give overarching civil rights to people with disabilities but remained fragmented in approach. Educational issues, for instance, are still dealt with under Education and Children Acts, not this act. However, it did establish that there is cross-party political and popular will to view disability issues from a civil rights perspective. As part of the package to support this act, there was also a practical alteration of Building Regulations to cover new-build construction of domestic dwellings requiring a visitability standard of new-build home accessibility. Part M of the Building Regulations 1991 was updated in 1998 and supported by Approved Document Part M: Access and Facilities for Disabled People, 1999 Edition. A further revision is currently in progress at the time of writing.

Social policy

The British context in which these civil rights issues are debated and the legislation framed is that of re-evaluating the social concepts of welfare and particularly the welfare state. There is a tension at the heart of this British style approach to welfare, between individual need and collective provision, between the safety net concept of collective responsibility from the early welfare state and the individualist, self-reliant ideology of the 1980s and 1990s (Jones, 2000).

The Labour government's approach from 1997 has been to promote partnership between welfare and voluntary agencies and for funding to be allocated within jointly planned commissions rather than by competitive contract tender as had been the case in the 1980s–90s' heyday of introducing business practice and competition into health and welfare services (DoH, 1997, 1998). However, the concept, if not the catch-phrase, of value for money continues with policies for evaluating local authority social services performance entitled 'Best Value'.

The central figures in planning of British social welfare from 1997 have been the stakeholders (DoH, 1997). The stakeholders are part of the idea that social problems cannot be tackled by any one agency alone. For example, it is a key health promotion concept that health is affected by lifestyle choices or lack of them, housing conditions, occupational hazards in employment or unemployment and educational opportunities or achievements. Thus the concept of partnership, which requires that agencies work together, arises from a view of the causes of social problems. However, the service users are one stakeholder among many.

Any change in social policy governing welfare provision has to meet the challenges of supporting members of a society in which the age balance is shifting, family structure and expectations are changing and in which the civil right of the individual is an increasingly understood and accepted social concept. Social policy in the form of law and its interpretation locally and nationally is tested in the courts through cases brought by individuals, or by lobby groups on behalf of individuals, against policies of welfare agencies which prevent people exercising or accessing those rights (Oliver, 1999). Professionals working in housing and social services agencies can become part of such cases, and occupational therapists are becoming more aware of their chances of involvement in such litigation either as a party in such a case or as an expert witness.

Working within a local authority context, it is also useful to bear in mind that the government of the day may or may not be reflected in the elected membership of the local authority. This can accentuate a difference in the local interpretation of policies fed down from the centre. While such differences and changes in policy may seem a little arbitrary and confusing to professional and user alike, it is part of the purpose of local authorities to reflect local differences and for local politics to modify national policies.

Some policy affecting local services is derived from global organisations by whose aims and agendas national government is influenced. The World Health Organisation Classification of Functioning, Disability and Health, which is a formative policy of how health and social care services structure their understanding of people with disabilities, has set itself a classification structure which does not accept terminology primarily of medical conditions and language. Instead, the categories for classification are body functions and structures, activities, participation and environmental factors (WHO, 2001). The underlying assumption is of an embodied person who will be active, participate fully in their social context and will find either support or barriers in the surrounding physical and social environment. This is a design which favours both the autonomy of the individual, by emphasising active aspects of life in which they may be self-directing, and also favours the values and practices of occupational therapists through concern for activities and participation (Chard, 2004).

Thus social policy and therefore local practice does shift over time as a new approach is taken on and an old one set aside. Keeping in touch with current social policy and identifying the current themes can help the practitioner understand how and why local policies are changing. It can even help the practitioner to be proactive in local change, ensuring that the voices of both users and professionals are heard by local decision-makers.

Postmodernism and the professions

Another of the current social policy debates is about the control of the professions: how do we demonstrate continuing proficiency in our fields, who checks that we are operating within the limits of our understanding and skill and who has the right to stop us practising?

Within the welfare systems, the NHS has introduced Clinical Governance (DoH, 1997; DoH, 1998) which requires within its quality remit that professionals demonstrate a currency of skill and knowledge. With the NHS Act 1999 comes a debate within the profession on how we will demonstrate to the new Health Professions Council our continuing competence to practise as therapists.

However, behind arguments about how to control professions, often carried out in glaring publicity, is a critique going back to Illich (1977) which questions whether the professions are as altruistic as they would like to think or whether they shape beliefs, events and policies to maintain their own prestige and status. It may even be that things are made worse for the users to maintain the professionals' ways of working.

Postmodern commentators go further. Taking the analysis particularly from the work of the French philosopher Foucault, a profession is a profession by virtue of its discipline. A discipline is both a body of knowledge or skill and also the way in which that knowledge and skill is exercised as power over others – the service users (Leonard, 1997). In exercising the discipline, the professional turns a disciplinary gaze upon the service user. Within this context, the user will give the professional information upon which the professional is empowered, legally and socially, to pass judgement. Is this true or false? Is this significant or insignificant? By this process the user is voluntarily subordinated – but, voluntary or not, it is still subordination. Within this context, the professional ultimately acts as an agent of state control answering questions such as: should this person be treated as mad? should this person receive this grant? how independent should this person be? From this perspective, it is understandably necessary for the state to exercise either immediate or remote control over what the professionals do.

Professionals taking a postmodern perspective on their work would promote the valuing of diversity and difference, support marginalised voices by ensuring that those who are shut out from access to social power get a hearing and work in smaller organisations nearer to the people served by them (Leonard, 1997). This is not far from the view of the disability movement:

> when confronted with decisions about scarce resources, professionals have usually sided with their management rather than with disabled people and our organisations in mounting political challenges to the unacceptability of such rationing. (Oliver, 1999, p. 379)

There is evidence that the profession is attempting to allow the user's voice a place in consideration of practice. For example, Winfield (2003) uses the opinion section of the *British Journal of Occupational Therapy* for a piece outlining his experience of helpful and unhelpful occupational therapy practice as it affected him in acquiring an adaptation. He is himself an academic and therefore perhaps a privileged voice and one which had the background more likely to allow him to be heard. However, this is the official journal of the British College of Occupational Therapists and thus his views reach and influence the full range of occupational therapists working in this country plus any overseas occupational therapists and researchers who use the journal as a reference source.

More systematically, Picking and Pain (2003) collected and analysed users' perspectives from 17 people who had experienced the middle range of complexity adaptations using focus groups. Alongside the process elements of their recommendations are professionals' qualities which the participants valued, including an understanding attitude, gentleness in encouraging decision-making and being sensitive to clients' needs in providing the right information at the right time to help decision-making progress.

A postmodern analysis of professionals says something to us about how we may act and relate to the users of our services as well as the organisations in which we could work.

Where, how and with whom we work in future depends on this kind of socio-political debate. Citizenship and rights are concepts currently being contested and so likely to remain debated issues for some time. Social policy and thus service provision will reflect the development and outcome of this debate.

More on socio-political perspectives

The socio-political perspectives related to occupational therapy practice are further considered in later chapters, including Chapter 2 ('The assessment process'), Chapter 3 ('The social model and clinical reasoning') and Chapter 4 ('Housing: the user's perspective').

Theory bases of occupational therapy

There is currently a good range of occupational therapy theories and models of practice to choose from in different areas of work and for different clients. It should be borne in mind that many, if not most, were not developed in this country or for these styles of housing service provision. Some models and their attendant assessment tools have been tested cross-culturally and some have not. In this section the generic problem-solving model will be considered together with models which have a concern for the physical environment.

Problem-solving process

Hagedorn (2001) sees problem-solving as a cognitive process rather than a theory. It is applicable to any professional intervention as the content of each stage is open to the decision of the individual using it. In a sense its usefulness lies in delaying the leap from seeing a problem to suggesting a solution: in closing to a decision too soon some other options may be missed.

Hagedorn describes problem-naming, problem-framing and problem-solving as the three parts of the process. Problem-naming is part of a client-centred approach which enables the client to identify the problem. For problem-framing, she gives the example (Hagedorn, 2001, p. 51) that a problem with going out of the house may be a problem framed as a mobility issue (quality of gait), a motivation issue (lack of interest) or an environmental barrier issue (steps). It is only when these two parts are complete that client-centred goal-setting can begin.

Problem-solving as part of the occupational therapy process begins with data collection. This may start with information given in referral or self-referral. It may be relevant to gather some background information at this early stage but often this will develop alongside problem identification, which will be made with the client and normally in the home setting. Making sure that there is agreement on the problem will allow the stage of identifying the desired outcome to be achieved more easily. It is also worthwhile ensuring agreement on what are the primary and what are the subsidiary problems. If there is a point in the process at which it becomes clear that not all the problems can be dealt with together, choices will be easier with the problem hierarchy already laid out. For the experienced therapist, cues may be identified which allow for a short cut to be made.

The desired outcome will often be expressed in terms of client function, for example 'The client will be able to go upstairs independently' or 'The client will be able to carry hot kitchenware without dropping it.' From identification of the desired outcome, solutions may be developed. This is the creative aspect to the model as the outcomes can only be as good as the ideas developed at this point. Some people are naturally gifted in being able to generate ideas spontaneously towards solutions, and others develop a good memory for the range of solutions they have used in the past or have seen others try out.

The range of solutions may be evaluated or appraised to choose the best fit for a client's wishes and function within a built environment. The extent to which options should be excluded from client appraisal because they are expensive or unwieldy is an ethical decision. Do you share an idea you know will never be funded and possibly disappoint the client and is it a waste of a client's time to pore over an idea which is technically difficult and hence unlikely to meet building professionals approval?

Having chosen an option, an action plan is developed and the solution implemented and any progress monitored. A final evaluation is made on completion, and, if another problem is identified at this stage, the cycle starts again.

The environment

'Environment' is a term with multiple usages for occupational therapists. While in daily usage for occupational therapists working in housing it tends to refer to the built environment, Hagedorn (1995, p. 94) considers its usage in occupational therapy theory in the sense of the cultural and social environment as well. This is not a major problem for practitioners as the object of work in housing is not just the built environment but the way that people live their daily lives within that built environment. This will automatically include issues of how activities are carried out, by whom, with whom and when.

Occupational therapy models and the built environment

Most, if not all, models of occupational therapy practice would claim to consider the built environment within their remit. However, it is clearer that the built environment is an intrinsic element rather than a bolt-on extra for those models which explicitly use the term 'environment' along-side 'person' and 'occupation' or 'occupational performance'.

For example, while Reed and Sanderson (1992) offer a detailed analysis of occupations and occupational performance skills, they suggest that changing the environment is only considered when enabling perform-ance in normal mode or changing that method of performance have failed. While changing the environment is a solution which tends to come after changing the performance mode, this approach to environment implicitly offers a rather negative view for therapists dealing with clients requiring environmental change. It also means most of the model will be geared towards intervention prior to this failure and so not particularly friendly to housing work.

In contrast, the Person-Environment-Occupational Performance Model (subtitled 'a transactive approach to occupational performance') works towards an optimum occupational performance by the person through establishing a congruence or at least a good fit between the triad of person, environment and occupation (Law et al., 1997, p. 93). Altering one aspect of the triad will affect the other two. The environment here includes the multiple meanings as discussed above but explicitly includes the physical environment as a particular consideration. The term 'transactive' seeks to capture an impression of the constantly changing nature of how people carry out their tasks over time within their environments. The model is Canadian and incorporates the Canadian Association of Occupational Therapists' guidelines on client-centred practice.

The Person-Environment-Occupational Performance Model (Christiansen and Baum, 1997, p. 87) also gives explicit validity to the consideration of the environment when assessing the person and their occupational performance. In this model the environment is seen as one of the extrinsic enablers of performance (Christiansen and Baum, 1997, p. 62) along with cultural, social and societal enablers. The demands the environment makes on a person acts by arousal (i.e. level of alertness) influencing whether and how an activity is carried out. The model is North American in origin.

There is still room for a model of occupational therapy practice which gives more consideration to the built environment. Meanwhile, the practising occupational therapist has increasing access to standardised assessments for community work. For instance, the 'Community Dependency Index' is specifically designed for assessment and outcome measurement in OT intervention (Eakin and Baird, 1995). The 'Housing Enabler' is a tool developed in Sweden which specifically assesses housing accessibility and has been shown to have a level of reliability. Its theoretical basis is explicitly linked to models which have a concern for the relationship between the person and the environment and the functional effect of altering environmental demand (Iwarsson, 1999). This tool has recently been extended to cover public buildings (Iwarsson et al., 2004).

Hagedorn (2000) distinguishes between a micro analysis of the near environment, as at a work station, and analysis of the used environment including a home and its curtilage, together with outside areas relevant to the person's valued activities whether paid or unpaid. She gives a detailed outline of the content of home assessments, the analysis of findings and making adaptations, all of which are pertinent and useful to occupational therapists working in the housing field. This is a comprehensive and relevant description of the process of assessment and making recommendations, not a model or a theory. It has practical application to professional practice rather than attempting a theory for that practice.

Finally, the emerging discipline of Occupational Science, which studies all aspects of human occupation, considers it important that these occupations should be studied within the contexts of their physical environments (Henderson, 1996). It may be that in future a taxonomy will be agreed to designate the range of an environment since an environment which is within what ergonomists would term the zone of comfortable or extended reach from the body is very different from that which a person needs to negotiate in order to reach the garage or the shops.

More on occupational therapy issues in practice

Occupational therapy issues in practice are further considered in later chapters, including Chapter 2 ('The assessment process'), Chapter 3 ('The social model and clinical reasoning') and Chapter 8 ('Ergonomics and housing').

Theory bases of design and construction

Ergonomics

This specialism has been interdisciplinary since its inception during the Second World War and may be defined as the 'science of fitting the job to the worker and the product to the user' (Pheasant, 1996, p. 5). Its uses range from design of whole working systems such as nuclear power stations, through equipment designs for industrial and domestic use and task designs to reduce health and safety risks right down to designs for better handles for a favourite coffee mug.

For the occupational therapist involved in housing, ergonomics assists with the design of domestic workstations (e.g. kitchen and bathroom) and analysis of the tasks undertaken in these domestic workstations.

An ergonomic task analysis consists of a breakdown of the activity under investigation into its component physical and cognitive parts, a bio-mechanical analysis of the forces affecting the body during the activity linked with the muscle action and effort required by the activity. The task analysis will take into account the physical environment in which the activity is carried out, including less concrete aspects such as illumination and temperature, and the general and specific risks inherent in the task. This analysis may have general application when shown to hold for an appropriate sample of a population, or have specific application for an individual when carried out as a single analysis. In the case of a specific application for an individual, the ergonomic task analysis is closely allied to an occupational therapy task analysis which is a core occupational therapy skill.

An example of analysis with wide application might be developing design principles for kitchen layout (Pheasant, 1996), for example the sequence of use of areas within the kitchen, for a right-handed person, tends to be from sink to work surface to cooking heat source to another work surface. The fridge, the sink and cooker form a triangle of most frequently used points for the general population. Goldsmith (1963) shows how this differs for a population with 'disability'.

Examples of analysis in the field with a single individual can range from the broad analysis of use of the home kitchen workstation by a particular person with a particular impairment and a particular lifestyle to the more intensive concentration on one aspect of an activity which is causing a problem, such as moving items from cupboard to work surface. Ergonomic analysis may also help give prominence to those aspects of task analysis sometimes ignored in the domestic setting, for example how does the quality, source and direction of light affect the task and how do signs, symbols and colours combine to allow the individual to control the task and equipment safely?

The design of furniture, storage and fittings for domestic environments is influenced by ergonomic theory and data. Occupational therapists find it helpful to have an awareness in particular of the branch of ergonomics concerned with identifying the measurements which will guide these designs – anthropometrics. All the equipment and furniture generally available on the market will be measured to these standards. So, for example, all working surfaces for tables and worktops will be set at a height which 95 per cent of the population will be able to use. The units for a wheelchair kitchen will likewise be set at a height which 95 per cent of the wheelchair-using population can manage. This 95th percentile rule allows an accommodation between the cost of production and the variety of need in a diverse population. Your particular client's measurements may or may not lie within the 95th percentile. The compromise between your client's needs and those of the rest of the family may not lie within this range, but to take the measurements outside of this standard is likely to raise costs as mass-produced kitchen units will need adapting.

Ergonomic principles will also underpin your approach to issues of moving and handling people (BackCare, 1999). In this case, you will be assessing hazards and risks inherent in and associated with the moving and handling task, looking to avoid hazards where possible and reduce risks. While moving and handling may appear to be a function of the client and carer rather than of the housing, environmental considerations affecting the moving and handling task are central to the assessment of risk and recommendations for practice. It is therefore necessary to consider issues of moving and handling alongside potential adaptations. For instance, where a person requires a hoist for their moving and handling needs, will the ground floor bedsit extension offer enough access for a mobile hoist to be used alongside the bed and any other fittings or does the extension structure allow for the installation of an overhead hoist for transfers from bed to toilet?

Here there is plenty of scope for occupational therapists to operate an ergonomic overview for their clients to obtain the best fit between a client's need, environment, equipment provided and moving and handling skills of formal and informal carers.

More on ergonomic design applied to space use

Ergonomic design applied to space use is further considered in later chapters, including Chapter 8 ('Ergonomics and housing') and a project integrating new technology into domestic buildings in Chapter 10 ('Smart technology at home').

Building, design and planning

Occupational therapists do not have a background in the building sciences: materials, design of buildings or building techniques. This is why they work within a team that includes building specialists such as surveyors, planners and builders. However, in order to enable them to formulate realistic options, a knowledge of building regulations and guidelines, reading and constructing plans, planning processes and timescales and a basic appreciation of how buildings are constructed is appropriate. This is not, perhaps, a coherent body of theory but more a collection of useful skills and knowledge related specifically to accessible design and dwelling adaptation processes.

Even with this knowledge and skill and a computer-assisted design package, an occupational therapist will not be able to take on the whole process. It does mean that they will share some language, skills and understanding with the building professionals which makes communication easier. Most importantly, it should also mean that the occupational therapist can ensure that the client has a clear understanding of the process and the real-world implications of plans and changes to plans.

More on building, design and planning

The legislation and regulations applicable to occupational therapists' work as well as the techniques of reading and constructing plans for adaptation, together with an outline of the planning process, are further considered in later chapters, particularly Chapter 5 ('Conveying information through drawing'), Chapter 6 ('Access standards: evolution of inclusive housing') and Chapter 10 ('Smart technology at home').

Theory base from health services

Biomedical approach

While the 'medical model' is seen in such a negative light from the socio-political perspective, knowledge of anatomy, physiology, medical conditions, the natural history of diseases, pharmacology and specific therapies, contraindications with conditions or treatments and medical risks are all used regularly as background to the work of occupational therapists in housing.

For example, if the condition which the service user has is deteriorating, what are the short- and long-term effects likely to be? Is it likely that this adaptation will be helpful to the service user by the time it is installed? For a musculoskeletal problem, what are the likely effects on the person if she uses this adaptation over time: will it reduce or increase pain, will it encourage joint distraction and deformity, will it aid mobility or leave the person at risk of falling? Will this rail aid that person in standing or is the pulling force required generating a cardiac risk? How does the medication affect this person's usual pattern of activity during the day and will a change in medication lead to a change in activity?

These are all common questions from everyday practice in housing. Since access to a medical record may not be possible or appropriate, and since rare conditions as well as common conditions are met with in community work, it is necessary for the occupational therapists to have both a firm grounding in biological sciences and medical conditions as well as a search/research facility to tap into at need.

Two final issues

Apart from theory bases, two issues affecting occupational therapists' practice will be considered. Care management as a tool for constructing the packages of support which people require alongside adaptations to live at home and evidence-based practice as a professional requirement for occupational therapy practice both have a formative impact upon the occupational therapist's work.

Care management

The majority of occupational therapists work with housing adaptations as part of local authority services. The adaptations are provided as part of a package of care that the client requires. How this package of care is developed, acquired, implemented and evaluated is the process of care management, and the responsible officer is a care manager. The occupational therapist concerned with housing may be a care manager in their own right or may have been brought in by a care manager.

The widespread implementation of care management as a system in the UK goes back to the comprehensive, national review of health and social care in the 1980s and particularly the White Paper 'Caring for People' (1989), which preceded the NHS and Community Care Act of 1990. The two simple ideas promoted in these White Papers were that people should be assessed for their individual needs rather than being fitted into existing services and that provision for these needs should come from a variety of sources and not just one monopolistic public service. As a consequence of these ideas, one person should be designated as responsible for identifying needs and purchasing but not providing the necessary services.

Envisioned as a means of offering flexibility and competition in service provision, care management has generated whole bodies of work on models of practice and evaluation of systems. Particularly, definitions of terms have been contested in academic, managerial and legal arenas. Some issues for the terms care, need and risks are considered below.

Care is a term with multiple meanings. We care for people emotionally and we provide care for our clients in return for direct or public payment. Relatives also provide care but do so within a different moral, ethical and emotional framework from paid carers. How many of these meanings of care does care management encompass?

Needs are not the same as wants, but when does one end and the other begin? This can become a real point of difficulty for a client in attempting to negotiate levels of care or the finished quality of adaptations. Needs can also become contentious in a time of financial stringency when the local authority attempts to curb its spending. A court challenge to Gloucestershire Council in 1995 by four elderly people whose home care had been withdrawn went from High Court to Appeal Court to the House of Lords. Gloucestershire was finally supported in its decision to take financial resources into consideration, and a further case has considered that the way needs are met can be influenced by financial resources (Langan, 1998; Mandelstam, 1999). These legal decisions have left local authorities with an anxiety about how needs should be expressed in writing and what this means in terms of liability.

Risk is another way of categorising a problem. The theory base behind, for example, assessment and management of risk for moving and handling the person being cared for, by the person or persons who are providing that care, may seem to have more to do with ergonomic than social care considerations. However, determining the risk of harm is a step back from identifying need (Langan, 1998) and may lead to differences in resource provision from a simple determination of need since risk takes into account implications for the carer and others affected by any such provision rather than focusing primarily on the person who has the need. Also, it could well be that a client has a clear view of their particular needs whereas identifying risk, as probability of harmful consequences, sounds a little more technical for a 'lay' person to argue and thus allows a professional claim to expertise in assessment. Risk assessment may be empowering if it allows the service user to take an informed decision on future action. It may also be disempowering, labelling the service user as especially vulnerable and even dependent (Malin et al., 2002).

Eligibility criteria and assessment process are means by which equity can be ensured across the service and/or managerial control can be exerted over resources through the kind of assessment made. Eligibility criteria here are the guidelines by which a person is judged able to receive some form of local authority social care. The criteria can be locally determined and related to risk assessment. The assessment process through which eligibility, or the lack of it, is judged tends to be guided by pro forma. There is evidence that the degree of user involvement is affected by the nature of the paperwork used (Langan, 1998) and that user input can be designed into the OT assessment process is evidenced in a study by Kent Occupational Therapy Bureau (Calnan et al., 2000), which showed a high rating by its service users on the dimensions of understanding problems and user input into decisions.

The occupational therapist's contact with the client will often be carried out within a process which is conceptually simple but practically complex. There may be real tension for the occupational therapist between the professional and ethical duty to support client autonomy (COT, 2001b), the duty to follow management procedure derived from the employment contract and their knowledge of available resources.

Evidence-based practice

Policies which currently drive services to demonstrate value for money and improvements in quality of service can be a lever for the implementation of evidence-based practice. Both service funders/providers and professional practitioners have a stake in ensuring that interventions have a demonstrable efficacy. Methodologies for collecting evidence have specialist theory bases of their own. All practitioners now need to acquire the basic skills for searching out, evaluating and implementing relevant sources of evidence for their own practice (COT, 2005, sections 5.4.3).

Little of our practice has been systematically researched, and the highest level of evidence acknowledged by the research community (Randomised Controlled Trials) is inappropriate as a medium for investigating many aspects of our work. A body of research-based evidence for OT using other methodologies is accumulating. Alongside evidence from research methodologies, OT includes non-research-based elements in its evidence base. These non-research elements may include the expertise of occupational therapists recognised in their fields, previous personal practitioner experience as well as clients' views and values (Bury and Mead, 1998).

At the level of the individual practitioner, evidence may also be gathered from OT assessments but thought should be given to the implications of using a standardised or non-standardised assessment: for instance Stewart found that in a comparison of a standardised against a non-standardised tool measuring severity of disability as gateway to services the non-standardised tool could disadvantage some client groups (Stewart, 1999).

Under registration requirements from the Health Act 1999, we will all need to demonstrate that we are keeping abreast of new developments as they become available. Planning to carry out Continuing Professional Development (CPD) activities will be essential. Within appraisal, learning requirements for CPD which fit both individual and service needs should be identified and provision negotiated. While provision may mean training, it could just as easily mean agreeing search and reading time, developing service evaluation projects or establishing a journal club within the service.

More on evidenced-based practice

Management approaches are further considered in later chapters, including Chapter 2 ('The assessment process'), Chapter 7 ('Housing adaptations and community care') and Chapter 9 ('Evaluation for service users and service performance').

Conclusion

Within this chapter, the theoretical background to the occupational therapist's work with housing has been outlined. While the range of bodies of work drawn from may seem wide, taking from several disciplines that which is useful to solving a specific client's problem is not out of keeping with the profession's pragmatic character. Human occupation is not a simple matter and will necessarily include more than one discipline's perspective. The trick is to ensure two things. First, that the theory borrowed is well understood and appropriately applied and, secondly, that the profession maintains its own unique viewpoint while using these approaches and is not fragmented and lost among them. Later chapters will pick up some of the issues raised in this chapter to address them in more depth and give them case application.

Key points

- *Socio-political approaches:* see Chapter 2 ('The assessment process'), Chapter 3 ('The social model and clinical reasoning') and Chapter 4 ('Housing: the user's perspective').
- *Occupational therapy approaches:* see Chapter 2 ('The assessment process'), Chapter 3 ('The social model and clinical reasoning') and Chapter 8 ('Ergonomics and occupational therapy in housing').
- *Ergonomics and building/design approaches:* see Chapter 5 ('Conveying information through drawing'), Chapter 6 ('Access standards: evolution of inclusive housing'), Chapter 8 ('Ergonomics and housing') and Chapter 10 ('Smart technology at home').
- *Care management and evidence-based practice:* see Chapter 2 ('The assessment process'), Chapter 7 ('Housing adaptations and community care') and Chapter 9 ('Evaluation for service users and service performance').

The assessment process

FRANCES HEYWOOD

In this chapter the complex process of assessment for housing adaptations will be addressed. A client-centred approach will be taken. Legal and moral rights will be considered alongside the difficult issue of defining needs. The meaning of home is reviewed, emphasising the importance of acknowledging the emotional investment people make in their homes, together with an understanding of how family life is influenced by specific design and decoration features. The particular needs of children are highlighted. Finally, service management context is examined together with approaches to assessment under limited resources.

Introduction

The process of delivering a satisfactory housing outcome for the disabled person begins with a sound assessment. Theory bases of 'socio-political approaches', 'occupational therapy approaches' and 'management approaches' discussed in Chapter 1 are the starting position. This chapter will illustrate the complexity of a process with all of these theory bases feeding into it. From socio-political approaches, the importance of a client-centred approach will be highlighted. From management approaches, the importance of interprofessional, cross-agency working and working within resource limits will become apparent. From occupational therapy approaches, the particular contribution of the occupational therapist's perspective will be considered.

Chapter 4 shows how a service user views the process of adaptation. This chapter will build on everything contained there to explore how, even amidst all the pressures of resource constraints, assessment can be client-centred, what that means and why we advocate this approach. And the starting point is to consider what assessment is.

Key elements of an assessment for housing adaptation

The first thing to remember is that it is the client's home, the client's life. What they want from the assessment is for the occupational therapist to understand what they need and the occupational therapist's skill in making a plan that will help them regain their home and resume their life. An occupational therapist's assessment for housing adaptation is a summing up of the problems experienced by the client in their home, the factors to be taken into account and a proposal for achieving the outcomes the client desires through alterations to the dwelling.

This means that an open mind and the ability to listen are as precious and important as knowledge and technical training. If imagination, foresight, creative thinking and negotiating skills are then added in, the result should be a very good assessment!

Why does the client need an occupational therapist? Because an occupational therapist knows about the progression of disabling impairments and knows what solutions to housing barriers exist and which are suitable for what problems. Why does an occupational therapist need the client? Because the circumstances of every person are unique.

Socio-political theories that underpin assessment

The concept of a client-centred approach to public services has evolved partly from a concern to respect difference while promoting equality of outcome, as explained in Chapter 1. It also fits with the concept of individual choice that is part of our consumer-orientated postmodern society.

The social model of disability

One important aspect of the provisions of the disabled facilities grant is that it reflects a social model of disability (see Chapter 3) and a moral theory of rights based on ideas of equality and justice. The objective of the legislation is to restore to the disabled occupant access to all the activities normally undertaken in a home. Assessment is an assessment of the barriers and of how they may be removed. The right is the right to the same enjoyment of the home as other citizens enjoy.

For managers in public services in Britain it has perhaps been difficult to accept this rights-based social model because of the long traditions within such services of seeing assessment as the assessment of the individual's problems, and provision as the benevolent distribution of 'welfare' to those whom they judge to be the most needy and most deserving. These views reflect no understanding of the structural causes of inequality or of the interdependence of assessors and assessed.

The concept of mutual dependence

There is a theory of mutual dependency which says, 'look more deeply and ask who is dependent on whom' (Dean and Taylor-Gooby, 1992, p. 2). The disabled person needs the occupational therapist, but the occupational therapist also needs the disabled person. For without disabled people occupational therapists would be out of a job, just as doctors would be if there were no sick people. This is mutual dependency, a useful idea to bear in mind.

Internationally supported rights of disabled people

The social model of disability and the idea of mutual dependency are two examples of ways of looking at the world that challenge the current assumptions about how the world works. Similar important challenges to thinking are to be found in ideas about human rights. The twentieth century saw a transformation in ideas of equality and justice, from a world where inequality because of class, gender or race (let alone other issues) was completely taken for granted to one where the right to equal treatment for the great diversity that is the human race is commonly asserted.

Some of the rights referred to in this book are rights in principle that have been stated in international declarations or conventions signed by various national governments. These do not make detailed provisions, but state a principle against which the behaviour of a government may be judged, or in some cases challenged in a court.

Some relevant points from these declarations and conventions are:

- The Universal Declaration of Human Rights 1948 and particularly Article 25.1 that:

  Everyone has the right to a standard of living adequate for the health and well-being of himself and of his family, including food, clothing, housing and medical care and necessary social services, and the right to security in the event of unemployment, sickness, disability, widowhood, old age or other lack of livelihood in circumstances beyond his control. (OHCHR, 1948)

- The European Convention on Human Rights 1950, which from October 2000 has been incorporated into domestic British law through the Human Rights Act 1998, states in Article 8.1 that 'Everyone has the right to respect for his private and family life' (Council of Europe, 1950).

People who believe their rights under these agreements have been abused may in some circumstances take their cases to court, including the European Court of Human Rights. This usually happens only after lengthy legal proceedings within the country of origin, where the suggestion that human rights have been infringed may be accepted or rejected by the judges to whom the case comes.

Internationally agreed rights of children

Children have internationally agreed rights too. Some of the relevant articles of the United Nations Convention on the Rights of the Child are given below. The United Kingdom has signed this convention, and occupational therapists carrying out assessments are thereby committed to consulting and giving due weight to the views of the children and young people they encounter. This applies to siblings as well as to the disabled child.

The United Nations Convention on the Rights of the Child 1989 states that:

> The child, for the full and harmonious development of his or her personality, should grow up in a family environment, in an atmosphere of happiness, love and understanding. (OHCHR, 1989, preamble)

and that:

> A mentally or physically disabled child should enjoy a full and decent life, in conditions which ensure dignity, promote self-reliance, and facilitate the child's active participation in the community. (Article 23 (1))

It also states that assistance:

> shall be designed to ensure that the disabled child has effective access to and receives education, training, health care services, rehabilitation services, preparation for employment and recreation opportunities in a manner conducive to the child's achieving the fullest possible social integration and individual development, including his or her cultural and spiritual development. (Article 23 (3))

And in considering the wishes of the child in relation to all matters affecting him or her, which would include adaptations, it sets the principle that 'A child who is capable of forming his or her own views' has 'the right to express those views freely in all matters affecting the child, the views of the child being given due weight in accordance with the age and maturity of the child' (Article 12).

Specific legal rights to adaptation

In addition to general human rights, disabled people may have legal rights to suitable adaptations enshrined in national legislation, which will, of course, vary from country to country.

In Britain a general right to adaptations was first assured in the Chronically Sick and Disabled Persons Act, section 2 (England and Wales,

1970; Scotland, 1972; Northern Ireland, 1978) which still applies. Some specific rights, however, are powerfully and clearly listed in the provisions of the Housing Grants, Construction and Regeneration Act 1996, section 23 which states the purposes for which grants *must* be provided.

(a) facilitating access by the disabled occupant to and from the dwelling or the building in which the dwelling or, as the case may be, flat is situated;

(b) making the dwelling or building safe for the disabled occupant and other persons residing with him;

(c) facilitating access by the disabled occupant to a room used or usable as the principal family room;

(d) facilitating access by the disabled occupant to, or providing for the disabled occupant, a room used or usable for sleeping;

(e) facilitating access by the disabled occupant to, or providing for the disabled occupant, a room in which there is a lavatory, or facilitating the use by the disabled occupant of such a facility;

(f) facilitating access by the disabled occupant to, or providing for the disabled occupant, a room in which there is a bath or shower (or both), or facilitating the use by the disabled person of such a facility;

(g) facilitating access by the disabled occupant to, or providing for the disabled occupant, a room in which there is a washhand basin, or facilitating the use by the disabled person of such a facility;

(h) facilitating the preparation and cooking of food by the disabled occupant;

(i) improving any heating system in the dwelling to meet the needs of the disabled occupant or, if there is no existing heating system in the dwelling or any such system is unsuitable for use by the disabled occupant, providing a heating system suitable to meet his needs;

(j) facilitating the use by the disabled occupant of a source of power, light or heat by altering the position of one or more means of access to or control of that source or by providing additional means of control;

(k) facilitating access and movement by the disabled occupant around the dwelling in order to enable him to care for a person who is normally resident in the dwelling and is in need of such care;

(l) such other purposes as may be specified by order of the Secretary of State.

This legislation is now reinforced in England by joint guidance from the Department of Health and the Office of the Deputy Prime Minister (ODPM/DoH, 2004). Similar guidance for Wales is contained in Circular 20/02 and in Northern Ireland there is a Good Practice Guide.

Any occupational therapist assessing for adaptations has a duty to ensure that the legal entitlements are met. In the past some managers in social services authorities have been unaware of the law because it was housing rather than social care law and generally dealt with by the housing department, a separate branch of the local authority. However, assuming to work to different aspects of law in different departments is a false distinction: the law is the law, and ignorance of the law is no defence.

Ombudsman rulings

In recent years in Britain there have also been rulings by the Local Government Ombudsman – the Commissioner for Local Administration in England (Wales and Northern Ireland have their own commissions) – concerning delayed assessments and the unsatisfactory provision of adaptations that have been judged to constitute maladministration. These have resulted in some quite large compensation payments to complainants and are an example of the serious enforcement of adaptation rights.

Theories of human need

Human rights cannot be proved, but have to be asserted and claimed. Such claims are based on the two key concepts of 'justice' and 'need'. All human beings should, in justice, have the right to whatever is needed to give them a chance of leading a reasonable existence. Needs therefore determine what human rights should be and the principle of justice decrees they are rights.

But who is to determine what is a need? Those who have struggled with the issue have come up with some helpful ideas. Doyal and Gough (1991) conclude that the two universal needs were for 'health' and 'autonomy'. Maslow (1970) talks of 'self-actualisation' being the ultimate human need. Both the idea of autonomy and the idea of self-actualisation seem highly relevant to assessment for adaptation, in addition to the need for health. They tie in closely with the theories of occupational therapy (see below). They are also both factors in determining the 'meaning of home' and help to show why taking it into account is so important.

Theories of the 'meaning of home'

Within the field of housing studies, there is a considerable literature on what is called 'the meaning of home'. This is of great importance to occupational therapists because it explains how adaptations may harm the clients they are supposed to benefit. The theory is that a person's home has layers of meaning for them beyond the simple, functional one of shelter from the elements. These ideas have emerged from the study of people writing about what their home means to them and from research among those who have lost, or are threatened with having to leave, their homes. One researcher has coined the word 'domicide' to describe the deliberate destruction of somebody's home (Porteous and Smith, 2001). Others have shown how older people who are forced to leave their homes and enter residential care, with no control over the decision, are likely to die soon afterwards (Seligman, 1975, p. 185). Adaptations, of course, are designed to help people remain in their homes and should not cause the death of the occupant or the destruction of the home. If badly done, however, they may severely interfere with how the person understands and responds to the changed home. This may be felt emotionally, like an assault. This is why it is important to reflect on what home means to people, and to be aware of vulnerable aspects when assessing for adaptations.

There is no one definitive list of all the positive meanings a person's home may represent. For children it is a place of nurture, play and growth; for adults it may be a financial investment. Other key aspects are shown in Table 2.1.

Table 2.1 Examples of the way in which unadapted housing may threaten aspects of the meaning of home and adapted housing restore them

Aspect of meaning of home	Example of this meaning threatened by unadapted housing	Example of the meaning restored by adaptation, as described by service users
A place of privacy	Person unable to reach and use a toilet, reliant on neighbour to come in and empty commode	'The provision of a self-contained w.c. has conferred dignity and privacy.'
A place of safety	Person in fear of falling every time they have a bath or shower	'The anxiety and worry about the possibility of child falling is reduced now he has his own level access facilities.'
A place where the dweller is in control and has autonomy	Person cannot move from room to room nor choose when to get up, bath or eat because of dependency on local authority carers	'The ability to gain access to the whole house is wonderful. No longer a prisoner.' 'It was the independence. Not always asking other people and being dependent on them.'
A nodal point from which you go out and to which you return	Person is trapped by steps and threshold, unable to leave the property	'Has helped social life – can now get out to go to daughter's in the car.'
A place to foster and reflect a sense of self	Person is finding it very hard to be 'labelled' as disabled and have this displayed to the world by 'different' sort of housing	'Kind guidance from occupational therapist. Kept as home. Normal kitchen as opposed to wheelchair.'

Table 2.1 continued

Aspect of meaning of home	Example of this meaning threatened by unadapted housing	Example of the meaning restored by adaptation, as described by service users
A place to foster the closest relationships	Dependence on family member for every aspect of bodily care creates an unwelcome imbalance in relationships	'The new toilet arrangements [*Clos-o-mat*] changed our relationship [husband and wife] as previously it was difficult.'
A repository of memories and of one's life story	Inability to manage might cause advisers to suggest a move	'They had come into the house when it was first built, had brought up three kids there and had a good view and marvellous neighbours; what more could they want?' (the adaptations had enabled them to stay)

Source: Heywood (2001).

These ideas about home have to be considered twice over by the occupational therapist in the process of assessment for adaptation. In the first place, the question is, 'Which of these meanings are marred for the applicant because of their disabling home?' The examples in Table 2.1 show how occupational therapists picked up these points and made sure they were covered in the assessment.

The second time they have to be considered is when adaptations are proposed, to ensure that the adaptation itself is not destroying some key aspect of the meaning of the person's home. Table 2.2 gives some examples of how this may happen.

Table 2.2 Ways in which adaptations may themselves threaten the meaning of home

Aspect of meaning of home	Example of this meaning threatened by insensitive or incomplete adaptation
A place where the dweller is in control of decisions	'I did not want the step lift or the through floor lift. I know I will need to use them but at the moment it is just an eyesore.'
A place to foster and reflect a sense of self	'The lifts would be a constant reminder of the client disability as not possible to put them out of sight.'
A means of displaying achievement and status to the outside world	'Builders destroyed the lawn and patio.'
A place to foster the family	'Works were done solely for Matthew. The rest of the family were left to use residual space.'

Source: Heywood (2001).

Needs specific to children

Although the disabled facilities grant is an excellent example of a provision based on human rights, it regrettably omits provision for the specific needs of children and does not reflect their rights as listed above.

Children are not just smaller adults. They have needs in housing that are different and additional to those of adults. These include the needs:

- *to develop*: a small child has to go through certain physical phases (rolling over, sitting, dropping things from a height) in order to develop mentally. Disabled children need these same experiences, but may need the environment altered in order to achieve them. In terms of social development, all kinds of experience, exploration and encounters with other people are necessary. We are shocked when we read of children tied to cots in neglected orphanages, partly because of the harm this will do to their development. We have to be sure we are not allowing a disabling environment to cause similar restrictions to children with impaired mobility.
- *to grow*: the growth that takes place between the ages of, say, 2 and 15 is unlike any other phase of human life other than the foetal stage. Assessment for children's adaptations must take this fact of changing height and weight (allowing for those cases where growth is likely to be restricted) and increasing maturity into account in a way that is not relevant to adult cases.
- *to play*: for most adults, the word 'play' has a frivolous connotation: the opposite of work. For children, play is a necessity, fundamental to their learning and growth. Part of the occupational therapist's task is to assess a child's access to play and to set out to remove the barriers or to provide positive assistance. The following examples from Heywood (2001) show the importance of remembering children's needs.

Assessments and children's needs

1. Development

The big benefit to him is that he can be more independent. Before he would have been stuck upstairs – and only able to indicate what he wanted by moaning. Now he comes into the kitchen with his mother – pulls the pots and pans out and generally explores in the way all children do. Of course, he is also getting older – but at a recent yearly review they were very pleased – he'd come on a great deal.

2. Spontaneous play

He has some friends around here and he likes to go outside the front when they are playing football and rugby. Before the adaptations, he had not been able to get out there alone. It had been a half-hour job to haul the chair through from the back and drag it through the house and he might only stay out there for ten minutes. Now he can take himself out whenever he wants to.

3. Non-allowance for growth

Whole adaptation is too small. No thought given to the fact that a child grows up (boy aged 14: adaptation specified when he was 4).

(extracts from interviews as part of the
research published as Heywood, 2001)

Theories of the nature of housing satisfaction

Even a fully accessible home may not work out for a family if the property is in the wrong location for them. This illustrates a very important aspect of housing theory relevant both to adaptation and to the option of moving. To be acceptable, a home has to meet the dweller's minimum standards in a range of areas. These include:

- cost (mortgage/rent, heating, upkeep, financial security);
- size (numbers and sizes of rooms, garden, parking space);
- location (including the view, access to work, school, family, the pub, safety from crime);
- comfort design and safety (steps, heating, sunshine, the look of the home);
- condition (roof, windows, wiring, freedom from damp);
- control (the freedom/responsibility of the householder to make decisions in the home);
- the ability to manage in the home.

In general, all these aspects of housing matter to nearly all people. The risk for disabled people is that professionals will assume that, because they are disabled, 'design' and 'ability to manage' are the only housing issues that matter, and that they may reasonably be offered any 'adapted' property regardless of its other characteristics. This is theoretically unsound, for disabled people may mind just as much about size, location, condition, control and cost factors (especially capital investment) as anyone else.

Client-centred assessment: other practical issues

Who is the client? Who should be assessed?

The disabled person will, naturally, be the first focus of the assessment, but in many cases it cannot end there, and the occupational therapist should also have in mind:

- Any other disabled members of the household
  That there may be more than one disabled person is a strong possibility in households of two older people. Case study 2.1 similarly shows how the needs of one child were at risk of being forgotten because of the more visible needs of his brother.

Case study 2.1
A family had two sons: one was in a wheelchair; the other, with no obvious physical impairment, had a degree of autism and also had epilepsy. When the assessment for adaptation was carried out, it focused on the needs of the child in a wheelchair. The parents later said that they felt the needs of their other child had not been well considered. He had no sense of fear and so was at risk of falling from an upstairs window, yet the windows and safety glass part of the adaptation had nearly been omitted. His needs were also forgotten in planning the implementation of the adaptation work. He was upset by the many disruptions to his routine, and the parents felt that the assessment in such cases could include advice on how to implement the work as sensitively as possible.

- Caregivers
  The person giving care may be at risk of injury and in urgent need of adaptation help. Research shows a litany of accidents and back injuries caused to caregivers by lifting and carrying. (See also Chapter 8, 'Ergonomics and housing'.)
- Other individual family members
  Research with the siblings of disabled children has shown how badly they too may be affected by unsuitable housing provision (Atkinson and Crawforth, 1995). If sleep is lost through disturbed nights, their health, growth and education will suffer. Where there is challenging behaviour, the rights of siblings to privacy and family life will also need protection through suitable adaptation of the home. Similarly, pregnant mothers who, for lack of adaptations, have to carry disabled children up stairs may be endangering the life of the unborn child.
- The working of the family as an organic whole
  Every disabled person who lives in a family is part of a unique living

organism of interconnected individuals that exists for mutual support and benefit. If the needs of the disabled person are considered in isolation from those of the family, there is a risk of destroying the benefits of care, help, love and support that the family gives.

Cultural sensitivity in understanding the family's needs

Among the major racial and religious groups that make up the multi-cultural society of Britain and other Western countries are some cultural patterns that affect how a home is used and what is important to those who live there. Jewish families need to be able to sit round a table for the Sabbath meal; families from the Indian sub-continent will traditionally have gatherings in their homes where men and women meet separately in different rooms. In some cultures it is almost impossible for an individual member to be understood except as part of the family: the family stands and falls together. If one child is invited to a birthday party, mother, siblings and grandmother may go as well.

It is very important for occupational therapists to find out about these broad factors, but such learning will never be enough by itself, because cultures are constantly on the move and because every individual family will interpret its culture differently. Being culturally sensitive is about more than just an awareness of broad cultural differences among migrant groups. There are indigenous cultures, sub-cultures and cultures unique to an individual family. (The Mozarts would need room for a piano.) In the assessment, therefore, the occupational therapist has to find out all they can about what is important to a family, so that the adaptation offered doesn't destroy something fundamental to the family's well-being.

There is no need to be concerned if an applicant sees there will be some benefit to the whole family as well as to the disabled person. The disabled person is a member of that family, and Case study 2.2 shows why such gains are to be treasured. The woman from southern Asia is quite open about the needs of the whole family and equally open in her obvious concern for the well-being of the older man and in her assumptions that the family will care for and include him in all that they do.

Case study 2.2
A woman discussing adaptations put in for her father:

'It was useful having the second toilet as their father often needed to use the toilet and that had been difficult if anyone had used the bath. While the adaptations had been for their father, the house was for all the family and they had to consider what their family needed both then and in the future.

> It is also easier to help their father in the downstairs shower and toilet room. It is usually his grandsons who help him shower, which he was happy with. He is close to the children and likes to be part of the family.'

When is an assessment complete?

Surely the assessment is over when the occupational therapist has visited the property, seen the situation and made recommendations about what is needed? This may be true in many cases. But in more complex cases the assessment will have to be more open. The family will want time to reflect and raise points they did not think of (or did not mention) at the first meeting. They may, after their official assessment meeting, get important advice about what is needed from someone who is an expert in their condition. As the work begins, builders may have sensible suggestions to make, and the occupational therapist should be ready to re-assess the situation.

Community occupational therapists are in great demand, and management will want them to achieve as much as possible in a single visit. But when the capital sums in large adaptations are considered, it has to be remembered that an extra two or three hours of an occupational therapist's time may prevent the mis-spending of thousands of pounds.

Case study 2.3
In one research area (Heywood, 2001), the managers of the adaptation process refused to send an occupational therapist to inspect when a client thought the adaptation was going badly wrong. The result was an adaptation costing £35,000 that was unusable. The authority subsequently paid out thousands more pounds to put the work right.

Management approaches to assessment for adaptations

At the highest strategic level, housing adaptations for adults and children should be seen as a means of supporting some of the government's core objectives: improving health, fostering education and employability, keeping people out of institutional care. In Northern Ireland a fundamental review of the adaptation system (NIHE, 2003b) involved health, social services and the housing sectors. The resulting report is an example of what is possible when joint approaches are taken seriously at all levels.

A range of strategic management approaches to assessment are possible:

1. How can we help whoever needs adaptation and secure the resources of people and capital to do so? (Finding Ways to say Yes)

2. How many people can we exclude from our service, or how can we limit capital outlay so as to stay within our allocated budget? (Finding Ways to say No)
3. Our first priorities are the targets set by all the monitoring bodies on which our service will be assessed.
4. We will employ competent professionals and leave them to make the judgements.
5. We will lay down strict rules covering every eventuality so as to be sure that the service we offer is uniform and equal and that all procedures are correctly followed by all staff.

The evidence concerning some of these approaches is that they are more likely to cause waste than lead to good outcomes for service users. Target chasing or control by rules may both have serious consequences for assessment. The desire to reduce waiting times may lead to rules that limit the time an assessment visit may take or stipulate that the whole assessment must be done in a single visit. Imposing this kind of economy on an occupational therapist's time has caused serious waste. Occupational therapists have to stand up to such pressures when they conflict with their professional standards.

Number 3 in this list should not be the driving force: the good performance indicators should flow from good service. Number 4 could serve number 1.

Care management

Chapter 1 described how assessment for adaptations for adults may take place within the larger framework of care management assessment, with its emphasis on assessing and prioritising a range of professionally determined, mainly functional needs. The move towards 'single assessment' approaches is important here. It does not mean that unqualified staff from other agencies could assess for major adaptations but it does mean closer working, some sharing of core information and letting others assess for and install minor adaptations. 'Fair Access to Care' (DoH, 2001) is another initiative within the world of care management that might be used to limit access to assessment for adaptations.

It is especially important in this context for occupational therapists to assert the social model of disability and to remember that adaptations are legal rights that cannot be set aside by local policies.

Risk assessment

Risk assessment is a core part of both care management and the work of environmental health officers, who in Britain are often tasked as officers responsible for handling the Disabled Facilities Grant and who also judge unfit housing. Occupational therapists can turn risk assessment to the advantage of clients by working with them to clarify the risks they face in their unadapted home. If this approach is linked to evidence and research, there will be opportunity to list not just risks of falling or admission to residential care, but also, for example, the risk of fire if only one accessible entrance is provided, or the risk of mental illness, especially depression.

Interprofessional or joint working

In Britain, community occupational therapists are often health-trained professionals, working for social services authorities to assess for a housing-funded grant administered by environmental health officers. In implementing adaptations, interprofessional working can scarcely be missed! But how relevant is it to the process of assessment?

The letter of the law in England, Wales and Northern Ireland divides the assessment process for disabled facilities grants into two stages: one to decide what is 'necessary and appropriate' and the other to consider what is 'reasonable and practicable' (Great Britain, 1996a, para. 24.3). Although the legislation is not explicit, it is common for this to be understood to mean that the occupational therapists will decide the first half and the housing or grants officers the second half. In simple situations this can be achieved in exactly this staged way. The occupational therapist says a stairlift is what is needed, and the housing professional, sometimes personally and sometimes via a stairlift company, checks the wiring and technical issues associated with the construction of the stairs, works out the likely costs and confirms the practicability. Both professions are necessary, for the housing professional will not know for which medical conditions stairlifts are unsuitable and the occupational therapist will not have detailed training in building requirements. From research (Heywood, 2001) it is clear those departments where there is mutual trust between the occupational therapists and the housing/grants officers and respect for each other's expertise work very efficiently in these straightforward cases.

In more complex cases the assessment will not be linear in this way but will require close interprofessional working, with dialogue and the exchange of information to come up with a workable assessment. Joint visits of occupational therapists and housing professionals, in dialogue with the individual or family, the builder and perhaps also including a planner, architect or structural engineer will be necessary to come up with an option that might solve the problem.

Which professionals?

Chapter 1 gives a list of some of the professionals with whom occupational therapists will work. To this list could be added:

• parents as professionals;
• disabled people as experts.

A 'professional' is normally understood to mean somebody who is paid to carry out a particular task. There is, however, another sense in which a 'profession' means a group of people with particular skills and expertise whose dedicated commitment to their main occupation permeates all aspects of their lives. Some parents of disabled children have made the point that by this definition they are professionals, expert in the needs of their own children and totally committed to promoting their well-being (McKeever, 2001). This may be a useful way of thinking about dialogue with parents. Research has shown how much such respect is valued and how productive it can be. Similarly, disabled people of all ages are the experts in themselves. Examples show how much it matters that this expertise is taken on board as part of the assessment and the waste that may follow if it is not.

The particular contribution of occupational therapists

What do occupational therapists bring to assessment that is special and different from the theoretical approaches of social work, nursing or housing? 'A holistic view' might be one answer, but professionals in other disciplines may well say they share this as a target. 'A particular set of skills linking physiology, psychology, knowledge of particular disabling conditions and knowledge of a range of remedies and therapies relating to impairment' is another answer that would hold true in many cases. But still misses the key theoretical point that originally marked occupational therapists out from other health-related professionals, which is their understanding of the importance of occupation to the well-being of human beings. This means that, when they are assessing housing needs, they go beyond the question of 'how can we help you survive?' to the question of 'what do you want to be able to do?' This is a practical point of great significance to the quality of assessment, particularly in times of resource limitation.

Joint working with clients

This is another area where communication and techniques for communication are vital. Show the family pictures of items you are suggesting, take them to see and try equipment, set up virtual reality visits and give them time to think.

The theoretical position is mutual respect for each other's areas of knowledge. Research shows clients have great respect for occupational therapists' expertise and gratitude for their guidance. People have even recorded their gratitude for something they initially did not want but which they were persuaded by the occupational therapist to accept. But it has to work both ways.

Case study 2.4
She felt that the toilet would have been better if it was a normal lower one rather than the high toilet as Myra tended to flop back onto it causing the seat to become loose and get damaged. If it had been lower, she would have been able to get up onto it from the floor where she tended to scoot around on her bottom. The mother did not feel that her views were listened to over this issue and she was the person who knew her daughter better than anyone.

Cross-agency working

In addition to their work across professions, occupational therapists are likely to be involved in plenty of cross-agency working. In theory, joint working to reduce overlap and provide a 'seamless service' underlines all government social policy. In practice, there are barriers that make it hard. Different agencies have different perspectives, talk different languages, fear that someone else may be after their money or taking their job, do not understand or respect the other agency and see them in stereotyped ways.

Best practice in assessment, however, happens when efforts are made to reject the stereotypes, get to know the other agencies and learn how they can be beneficial.

Table 2.3 gives an idea of the different ways in which different agencies may be involved in assessment for adaptation. What a daunting list for the new occupational therapist! Imagine what the client feels like!

Case study 2.5
'There sometimes seemed to be so many people at the door the family just said, "Come in", and let them walk around and get on with it.'

One key message for any occupational therapist committed to client-centred working is not to see agencies who offer support to a client as a threat. Be confident, see what a benefit it is to the client and work with, not against, the flow.

Table 2.3 Inter-agency work in assessment: some examples using British organisations for health, welfare and housing

Role in assessment	Agencies who fill this role	Added value resulting
Sources of initial referral	Social services adult teams Hospital Trusts (hospital-based occupational therapists) Primary Care Trusts (health visitors, district nurses and GPs)	Useful relevant information, saving time for the occupational therapist
Referral and main source of funding	Local authority housing departments Local authority private sector grants departments	Will also help if other building work needed
Referral and some funding to offer	Specialist social services teams for disabled children: Housing officers from housing associations, also known as RSLs (Registered Social Landlords)	Knowledge of family Some RSLs fund their own adaptations and want only the expertise of the occupational therapist
Advocacy/support to client	Home Improvement Agencies Disabled Persons Housing Services Other charities who offer a service of advice and support (for example Age Concern or Contact a Family	Help to occupational therapist in giving time to listen to client Benefits advice and help with charitable fund-raising may also be offered Home Improvement Agencies and Disabled People's Housing Services may also offer support to look at moving options
Source of specialised occupational therapist knowledge	Charities that employ specialist occupational therapists to advise and support people with particular conditions Paediatric occupational therapists	Offer challenge, stimulus and key specialised knowledge about problems and solutions
Source of specialised technical knowledge	Local authority planning departments Private companies supplying items of equipment Architects or surveyors employed as 'agents' for the design and overseeing of an adaptation Experienced builders and HIA technical officers	Also offer challenge, stimulus and key specialised knowledge about solutions

Working with resource limits

There is nothing odd about working with resource limits. Most of us live our whole lives making choices between different things we would like to have and do because we do not have unlimited funds. We are used to weighing up whether it is better to go for cheap and short lived or good quality and much more expensive. We know that there is such a thing as 'false economy' and that it is pointless to buy a garment for a teenager, however sensible and functional it may be, if wearing it would destroy their 'image', because they won't wear it. Most people, if cash is limited, can accept the reality of the situation and make choices within a budget. But some things cost what they cost.

The complication with adaptation expenditure is that the money involved may be partly or mainly public money and that it is not in the direct control of the person needing the adaptations. Does the occupational therapist then see themselves as the champion of the disabled person or as the guardian of the public purse? Or do they see themselves chiefly as the employee whose managers have given instructions and laid down guidelines that must be followed? Often they will be playing all these roles at once, but it may be helpful to spell out some principles to help think things through at the time of assessment (see Table 2.4).

Table 2.4 Principles for working in a time of resource limitation

Principle	Carrying out the principle
Client's needs first	This is not so hard to hang onto when the occupational therapists' professional code of conduct is remembered. There is simply no point in doing an adaptation if it does not meet the needs of the client as perceived by themselves. Your job is to serve the client. But this is not just a question of professional ethics. There is a growing 'evidence base' that not heeding the views of the client leads to serious waste (Heywood, 2001, pp. 24–7). There are therefore sound financial and managerial reasons for strengthening, not weakening, the client-centred approach when resources are tight
Give options – leave control with client	So what happens when the client wants a downstairs toilet but you feel their needs to reach a toilet can be adequately met by the provision of a stairlift? You judge that this would be better because it would be less expensive and so leave more adaptation money available for others waiting. The answer is that if you impose your solution you may seriously disempower the person you are trying to help and possibly cause depression. So first you have to bear in mind that not only do they have a need to reach the toilet but they also need to retain the meaning of their home and sense of self. The way out of this is to return the control over the decision to the client by offering options. Would they be willing to contribute the difference in cost between the stairlift and the downstairs WC? Would they rather move? Would they be interested in seeing different types of stairlift? What other choices could there be?
Discretion must not be fettered	This key legal principle applies to all British local authorities and the joint guidance 'Delivering Adaptations' (ODPM/DoH, 2004) spells out what this means for the assessment of adaptations. Even when

Table 2.4 continued

Principle	Carrying out the principle
Discretion must not be fettered (*cont'd*)	resources are tight, local authorities may not make blanket policies that limit legal entitlement and prevent professionals involved in assessment judging each case on merit. They are not, for example, allowed to say, 'no grant over £14,000 will be considered' when the legal limit is more (£25,000 in England at the time of writing) or 'assessment for bathing adaptations will only be considered if there is a medical need to bath'. These (and other similar practices designed to manage resources) have been common but are unlawful
Know about all sources of funding and be prepared to 'ask for more'	When one budget runs out, there may be another. The occupational therapist who is convinced of the validity of an assessment that costs more than is available has to be prepared to go looking for other sources. Councillors will sometimes vote more money if a good case is made. Some health bodies support Home Improvement Agencies; the Housing Corporation has funds for expensive RSL adaptations; Disabled children are entitled to help under section 17 of the Children Act; Social Services have duties to adults under the CSDP Act 1970; there are schemes to help fund improved heating and there are charities and HIAs who will help clients apply. There may well also be new cheap loan schemes on offer in local authorities
Keep records	In accordance with the code of professional practice, occupational therapists should keep records of unmet need. This is the most powerful way of building up evidence of the need for more resources. Such information is like gold. One useful approach may be to turn risk assessment to advantage by carrying out a risk assessment of what will happen to a client if adaptations are not carried out

The Code of Ethics and Professional Conduct for Occupational Therapists states that 'the occupational therapist has a prime duty to the client' (COT, 2005, section 4.5.1). It also offers specific guidance about the duty of advocacy, duty to record unmet need and duty to bring resource and service deficiencies to the attention of employers (section 3.3). No one expects a doctor to break the Hippocratic Oath for the convenience of hospital administration (although pressure is certainly sometimes brought to bear) and occupational therapists may similarly assert the rules of their profession and expect to have them respected. It is not that a good occupational therapist must be constantly in conflict with an employer with different priorities but that when the crunch comes he or she must be clear where the first loyalty lies. Negotiation and compromise may well be necessary but, bearing in mind the concept of interdependence, the principle that the client comes first must not be abandoned.

Evidence-based practice

The principles of evidence-based practice and the obligation on occupational therapists to practise it are spelt out in Chapter 1 and are crucially relevant to practice. Using evidence in this practical area is not simply reading the latest study on service delivery or environmental design but valuing and incorporating therapists' and families' experiences as Case studies 2.6 and 2.7 show.

Case study 2.6
'Mother insisted on the design, as the importance of this was stressed by other families in the same position she knew about.'

Case study 2.7
'Look at the wider environment and village facilities such as schools, bus service, shops, post office. Are there any hills? Is there access to their friends' houses? Are there hedges with thorns which can cause wheelchair punctures? The child's needs change but the building can't change. Look at temporary changes. Also, before any adaptations commence, have an initial consultation as a team (everybody involved in the process) communication.' (Comment from parent asked to suggest improvements to the adaptation service)

The mother in Case study 2.6 was making an evidence-based input into the assessment: the evidence was the crucial experience of other families with a similarly disabled child. Case study 2.7, which is feedback from a parent, shows the value of a family's experience as evidence. Similarly, occupational therapists who use the experience of specialists, builders or home improvement agencies are all practising evidence-based work.

Conclusion

Case study 2.8
'The main point is to get it right at the beginning, at the assessment stage. The assessment needs to be done properly, not just for now but for the future as well. It would save a lot of time for everyone, because the grants officer and builders can only work to the recommendation given.' (adaptation recipient, 2000)

This chapter has tried to show some of the theories and ideas that lie behind the apparently simple business of assessment for a housing adaptation. It is not always so complicated. Many people with an awkward front step will be happy to have a grab rail to make it safer without any need for a profound understanding of wider issues. And yet the spirit in which things are done is always important and can enhance or reduce the value of the adaptation by leaving people feeling diminished or empowered.

When it comes to larger adaptations, however, the theories and principles of assessment become really important and can make the difference between life-enhancing effective adaptations and disastrous ones. Is the adaptation seen as an act of charity or of justice and legal entitlement? What are the internationally agreed rights of adults and of children? Who is dependent on whom? How should theories of the meaning of home impact on assessment? Whose needs should be assessed?

In considering these issues, therapists and managers alike will want to consider the evidence base that underpins their practice. And the role of management approaches in assisting good assessment is also crucial. Is their joint-working and cross-agency working based on real mutual respect and skill pooling? Do the ways of managing limited resources still reflect a client-centred approach?

Finally there is the discipline and profession of occupational therapy itself. The code of professional conduct offers clear guidance on priorities and the problem of restricted resources; the theoretical approaches of the discipline encourage therapists to understand assessment in the context of everything that makes a human being human. A good occupational therapist will never stop thinking and learning. They will bring to the process of assessment the key ingredients of their own training and knowledge, their ability to listen and their skill in valuing and using what other professionals and agencies have to offer.

Key points

- Good assessment will begin from the service user's perspective and an understanding of what that person wants to be able to do, how that person lives in this specific building with this family, their practices and beliefs.
- The home is not simply a built environment but a source of emotional meaning and support which can be damaged by insensitive adaptation.
- Children have specific needs which should be recognised.
- Good joint working between professionals, agencies and family is essential for a satisfactory result.
- Working with limited resources, there are principles which may be followed by occupational therapists.

CHAPTER 3

The social model and clinical reasoning

SUE PENGELLY

All occupational therapists that carry out adaptation work are involved in making complex decisions which have major long-term effects on people's homes. These decisions need to be made in partnership with disabled people and based on sound clinical reasoning. This chapter offers the reader the opportunity to deepen their understanding of both the social model of disability and clinical reasoning and to consider how these can impact on:

* *understanding housing problems;*
* *the relationship between professionals and disabled people;*
* *solving housing problems.*

Readers are encouraged to use this understanding to help implement the social model within their own practice and to be able to enhance their clinical reasoning within this complex area of practice. A deeper understanding of disability and clinical reasoning can help the development of a firm evidence base for use within this setting.

Introduction

Client-centred, social model thinking does not stop with assessment. From a sound assessment the process of delivering a satisfactory housing outcome for the user continues with sound clinical reasoning and decision-making. Theory bases of 'socio-political approaches' and 'occupational therapy approaches' discussed in Chapter 1 inform clinical reasoning in housing work. This chapter will illustrate how the social model and client-centred approach can be integrated into therapists' clinical reasoning throughout the problem-solving process and during the implementation of recommendations.

This chapter does not seek to provide a set of ground rules by which to act, but rather to encourage a deeper level of understanding of both disability and clinical reasoning which can be manifested by OTs working within housing.

It has been recognised that OTs working in housing engage in complex clinical reasoning and decision-making (Munroe, 1996). If the reader has any experience in this area, a brief review of their own practice is likely to confirm this. It is important for OTs within housing to be mindful of their own clinical reasoning since the decisions they make affect homes where people live. Both for the profession and for the sake of people who live in these homes it is important for OTs working in this setting to develop their ability to think rationally, creatively and in collaboration with people with disabilities. A greater understanding of clinical reasoning and how this is influenced by differing models of disability will help to clarify their thinking. This is an important step towards providing a clear evidence base for this area of practice. It is especially timely in the UK with a move towards greater integration of community working which will result in a broader range of OTs being responsible for undertaking adaptation work beyond those in the traditional social services setting. Throughout the chapter the phrase 'OTs working in housing' is used to encompass all OTs involved in adaptation work, irrespective of their work setting.

In simple terms, clinical reasoning is the thinking underlying clinical practice (Higgs and Jones, 2000). It is where theory and practice meet: where judgement is put into action, and where action generates knowledge (Mattingly and Fleming, 1994).

While undertaking an assessment, OTs aim to identify what occupational problems individuals have and then to understand what may have caused those problems before they can attempt to solve them. This reflects the two stages involved in problem-solving which are – *problem representation* (how the problem is understood and goals for action) and *problem-solving* (how the problem can best be overcome) (Robertson, 1996). Throughout this whole process partnership working should be maintained. This chapter considers these issues within the following three sections.

- *Understanding the problem:* Different ways of understanding disability, including the medical and social models of disability and OT models of practice; each have distinct consequences for housing practice.
- *Relationships between professionals and disabled people:* The medicalisation of disability and the socio-political approaches each influence the relationship between professionals and disabled people. OTs who are serious about working in partnership with disabled people need to understand the power dynamics inherent in that relationship and their impact on decisions made within housing.
- *Solving the problem:* OTs involved in making collaborative decisions to overcome housing problems employ three different types of reasoning.

These can be used through reflective practice to ensure that client-centred, social model intervention is carried out in housing. They are:

- theory-based reasoning (e.g. social model theory – to overcome barriers);
- meaning-based reasoning (understanding the client, their home and family);
- pragmatic reasoning (recognising the context in which OTs work).

Understanding the problem

In real world practice, problems do not present themselves to the practitioner as givens . . . When we set the problem, we select what we will treat as the 'things' of the situation, we set the boundaries of our attention to it, and we impose upon it a coherence which allows us to say what is wrong, and in what directions the situation needs to be changed. (Schön, 1983, p. 40)

Models of disability and OT models of practice will both influence how problems are understood by OTs working within housing.

Models of disability

The medical and social models present opposing views of disability. While one focuses on a biomedical perspective, the other draws upon socio-political theory to provide an understanding of disability. The fundamental differences between the two show divergent ways of framing the problem of disability which will affect the subsequent problem-solving process.

The medical model

The medical model is based on an understanding of how the body works. It will be explained using terminology which has subsequently become outdated. It argues that when a medical problem damages the body (impairment) this affects the functioning of individuals (disability), and ultimately their role in society (handicap). This is illustrated in Figure 3.1.

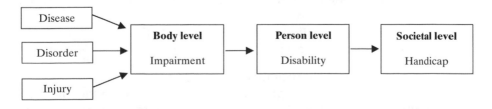

Figure 3.1 Medical Model.

Within the medical model, the problem of disability is firmly located within the individual. It is caused by an impairment and results in restricted participation in society. The impact of this way of understanding disability will be considered in relation to Case study 3.1.

Case study 3.1: Mr Smith
Mr Smith suffered a CVA five months ago and received several weeks of inpatient rehabilitation. Despite this input, he has a permanent right hemiplegia. As he is wheelchair dependent, he is unable to get in or out of his house, which has steps on access (see Figure 3.2).

This understanding of the problem impacts on the problem-solving process. Once Mr Smith's acute medical problem had been stabilised, the hospital OT used a neuro-developmental approach which aimed to maximise his recovery and reduce his resultant disability. Owing to Mr Smith's limited recovery, a functional rehabilitation approach is now needed to compensate for his remaining lack of functional ability.

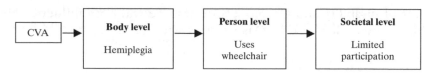

Figure 3.2 Medical Model applied to Mr Smith.

The social model

In contrast with the previous model, the social model locates the causal problem of disability as lying within a society which fails to meet the needs of disabled people (Oliver, 1996). Adjustment is therefore a problem for society, not for individuals. This shift in understanding disability is so fundamental that it has been presented as a paradigm shift (Oliver and Sapey, 1999).

Three main types of social barriers can be identified which disable people:

- *Attitudinal*: Prejudice and discrimination as the result of being labelled abnormal.
- *Organisational*: Segregation and limited opportunities in education, employment, housing etc.
- *Built environment*: Built for the able-bodied therefore presenting numerous barriers to people with impairments.

Figure 3.3 graphically illustrates this.

Social barriers disable people with impairments by restricting their opportunities to participate equally in society. Physical impairments are

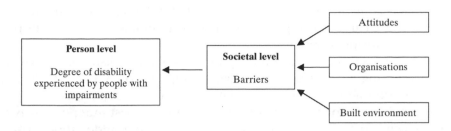

Figure 3.3 Social Model.

not ignored, but are taken as given, rather than being identified as the underlying cause of the problem.

Case study 3.1 revisited: Mr Smith revisited

Mr Smith is a wheelchair user and since his return home from hospital he has rarely left his house due to the steps. This has severely limited his opportunities to participate in his community (see Figure 3.4).

Once the problem of disability has been framed differently then the focus for problem-solving also changes. Mr Smith is visited by an OT who is familiar with his medical history and aware of his impairment but recognises that it is the steps to his home which are disabling him. The focus is on the removal of barriers.

In terms of the medical model, adaptation work was the last resort, to be tried when all else had failed. From the social model perspective, housing is an essential area in which OTs can work together with disabled people to remove disabling barriers.

The case study can be revisited with this alternative way of understanding disability (see Case study 3.2).

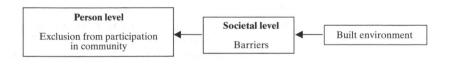

Figure 3.4 Social Model applied to Mr Smith.

OT models of practice

Beyond models of disability, OT models provide OTs with a conceptual lens through which to view and understand problems. These encapsulate the value of occupations, and a holistic and humanistic approach to problem-solving. For the purposes of this chapter, the Canadian Model of

Occupational Performance (CMOP) (CAOT, 1997) will be referred to as it provides a clear visual representation of OT thinking and actively promotes client-centred practice.

The Canadian model graphically illustrates the holistic nature of OT by presenting a dynamic inter-relationship between individuals and their environment through their engagement in occupations. The person and the environment are not understood to exist independently of one another, nor is the relationship between them understood in simple terms of cause and effect, as was the case with both the medical and social models. Both models of disability could be located within a single section of the Canadian model. The medical model pays exclusive attention to the individual, while the social model only focuses on the environment. When challenged about the limited theoretical focus of the social model, Oliver (1996) argues that it was not developed to provide a total explanation but rather to aid understanding and help overcome oppression and as a practical tool to produce social and political change (Oliver, 2004). While the social model is not sufficient to replace the holistic perspective embodied in professional models, it is invaluable to help understand the significant impact that the environment has and to balance the former tendency to locate problems within the individual.

OT is also founded on humanistic ideas, which encapsulate the concepts of individual worth and free will and form the basis for client-centred practice.

> CMOP portrays persons as spiritual beings who are active agents with the potential to identify, choose and engage in occupations in their environment. (CAOT, 1997, p. 3)

In contrast, the social model focuses on the impact that external factors have upon people, and its proponents have asserted that the humanistic belief obscures the social causes of disablement and diverts attention away from the social structural constraints upon human action (Abberley, 1995). The Canadian model has suggested that people are free within certain limitations and that individuals interact with their environment rather than are determined by it. From an OT perspective, acknowledging the abilities of individuals does not exclude recognising the impact of social barriers.

OT is recognised to be a very broad-based profession which blends a wide range of theoretical bases (including medical and social sciences) and seeks to use these in a way consistent with OT philosophy. While recognising the impact of social forces, it is important for OTs to also maintain their client-centred and holistic approach to understanding problems.

Relationships between professionals and disabled people

Understanding disability from a socio-political perspective rather than from a biomedical one will have a significant impact on the working relationships between professionals and people with disabilities. To understand this, some underlying ideas will be explored before considering their impact on practice through a case study example.

Medicalisation of disability

The medical model has become such a dominant way of understanding disability that its influence has passed beyond the bounds of medicine. Three other views of disability serve to demonstrate the pervasive influence of the medicalisation of disability.

- *The psychodynamic model*: The major task of the professional operating within this model is to adjust the individual to their particular disabling condition, including both changes in body image and loss of social roles/opportunities (Oliver and Sapey, 1999).
- *The personal tragedy model*: The medicalisation of disability focuses on the loss of a 'normal healthy body', which results in perceiving people with disabilities as being victims who are dependent on help from others. It has been argued that this model has influenced the development of both social policy and professional attitudes (Oliver, 1990).
- *The administration model of disability*: This model concentrates on the relationship between disabled people and service providers. Once disabled people are viewed as dependent victims, it follows that they will need other people to assess and provide for their needs (Finkelstein, 1993).

For the purpose of this chapter the term 'medical model' will continue to be used but the wider implications of the medicalisation of disability will be held to be implicit in this terminology. This wider understanding of disability will affect the relationship between professionals and disabled people, which is demonstrated in the following hypothetical case study.

Case study 3.2: Mrs Pimms
An OT carried out a visit to Mrs Pimms, a 42-year-old woman with multiple sclerosis (MS) who had requested the installation of a stairlift. No other functional problems were revealed during the initial interview. An enquiry about her physical symptoms revealed that fatigue and occasional visual disturbances were her main problems at present. However, the OT

understood the degenerative nature of MS and decided that it would not be appropriate to recommend a stairlift, owing to future safety issues. She explained to Mrs Pimms that she did not meet the criteria for a stairlift and proposed that a wheelchair-accessible vertical lift be installed instead. She arranged for an expert to visit the house to check that this would be structurally possible. Mrs Pimms commented that she did not know much about lifts and expressed concern about how it would look. The OT told her not to worry as everything would be sorted out for her and she was bound to get used to it in time. As the expert, the OT took the lead in the decision-making process and the client complied with the decisions taken.

Socio-political approaches

In contrast to the medical model, socio-political approaches consider the broader social context rather than explain things in purely individualistic terms. The two key ideas to be considered here are the social construction of disability and the recognition of rights.

Social construction of disability

Interpretive sociologists shifted the focus away from inherent characteristics of an individual towards social interactions by emphasising the importance of social values and attitudes in the experience of disability. The study of deviance and labelling theory were especially significant in the development of the concept that disabled people are not 'normal' (Abberley, 1993). Shearer (1981) argues that, if society could exclude people by labelling them, a change in social attitudes could re-include people who had previously been considered abnormal; left-handed people are rarely considered 'sinister' nowadays. These ideas have influenced the current promotion of valuing diversity and social inclusion and form the basis for disability awareness training. If the problem is understood to be the attitudes of individuals, the solution is to change these and thereby overcome the disabling influences in society.

Demanding rights

Abberley (1993) traces the development of thinking about disability and argues that it has moved through three stages, each of which had its own associated solution.

1. the individual models – with the call for individuals to change;
2. the social construction of disability – with the call for social attitudes to change;
3. the political arena – where disabled people demand their rights.

The redefinition of disability as being socially constructed brought discrimination issues into the foreground (Barnes, 1991). Existing inequalities and experiences which had formerly been regarded as inevitable consequences of impairment were reconceptualised as unacceptable discrimination which could be overcome by disabled people demanding equal rights (Abberley, 1993). If disability was socially caused, then it could be overcome through political struggle for social change (Oliver, 1996). Societal structures needed to change so that people with disabilities could function as full citizens with equal opportunities (Neufeldt, 1999).

> Largely through the efforts of disabled people themselves, disability has been relocated into the arena of human and civil rights. (Clements and Read, 2003, p. 93)

Making use of these socio-political approaches requires a change in mindset away from treating people like patients in hospital towards working with citizens in the community. This clearly impacts on the relationship between professionals and disabled people.

Case study 3.2 – revisited: Mrs Pimms revisited
An OT visited Mrs Pimms who explained that managing the stairs was her current concern. Having gained an understanding of how MS affecting Mrs Pimms, the OT discussed the advantages and possible future disadvantages of a stairlift with her. As a member of the MS Society, Mrs Pimms had talked with other people about stairlifts and the OT shared her own experience of previous adaptations. Possible alternatives were considered and literature on lifts was supplied but it was also recommended that Mrs Pimms should see one in situ so she could make a fully informed decision. It was agreed to check the structural suitability of the property to help make the final decision. Mrs Pimms was fully informed and was actively involved in the decision-making process.

A shift in power relationships and the role of professionals

Social model thinking introduced the idea that it was politically naive to consider relationships between professionals and disabled people without a clear understanding of the power dynamics involved. If the problem-solving process remained in the hands of the professionals, then assessment, planning, intervention and evaluation could all serve as barriers to the self-determination of disabled people (Priestley, 1999). Problem-solving under the medical model where the 'professional knows best' is in direct conflict with the aim of the social model.

These ideas present a challenge to health and social care professionals to consider adapting their role to adjust to this shift in the power relationship. Their future role should be based upon the understanding that they are a resource to be drawn upon to provide expertise and knowledge where it is useful to disabled people. OTs can focus on analysing the problems identified by the client and offering them a range of solutions (Hawkins and Stewart, 2002). The emphasis of practice should be on the identification and removal of barriers in partnership with disabled people (Picking, 2000). Within housing, OTs need to move towards a more consultative role which recognises the right of disabled people to be involved as partners (Nocon and Pleace, 1997).

Solving the problem

Along with other professionals, OTs have shifted from attempting to solve problems by thinking like rational technicians to becoming reflective practitioners (Schön, 1983). This has occurred due to the increased recognition of the complexity of the problem-solving issues they face within professional practice.

Literature relating to how OTs carry out clinical reasoning suggests that practitioners do not simply adopt one way of thinking, but instead use 'multiple modes of reasoning' (Mattingly and Fleming, 1994; Schell, 1998). This enables them to apply differing types of reasoning to the varied aspects of the problems encountered in practice. Research within health concluded that OTs operated a 'three-track mind' (Fleming, 1991), and this has since been found to be applicable to OTs within housing (Munroe, 1996; Medhurst and Ryan, 1996a; Fortune and Ryan, 1996).

Clinical reasoning is the fundamental process used by practitioners to plan, perform and reflect on client care (Schell, 1998). However, despite the importance of their decision-making, experienced OTs often find it difficult to articulate the thinking processes which lie behind their problem-solving as these often occur at a tacit or subconscious level (Mattingly and Fleming, 1994). A greater understanding of clinical reasoning can help to make these processes more explicit. In practice this helps to ensure decisions remain client-centred, and enables OTs to justify their decisions to a broad range of people including care managers, grants officers, fund holders, elected members and complaints investigators. Overt clinical reasoning is also invaluable in helping expert practitioners explain their reasoning to students and novices, who might otherwise remain unaware of the complexity of the decisions taken. Regular supervision with another OT who is experienced in housing can be an effective way of becoming familiar with articulating the clinical reasoning process.

An historical perspective on clinical reasoning reveals that it has paralleled developments within the profession (Chapparo and Ranka, 2000). While the medical model prevailed, clinical reasoning was focused around the application of professional theory to practice situations. It was then acknowledged that this theory-based reasoning did not take account of the client's perspective (Mattingly and Fleming, 1994). Within the climate of client-centred practice, an alternative meaning-based reasoning was identified (Mattingly, 1991a). More recently, there has been an increased recognition that clinical reasoning is not context-free but occurs within a socio-political and economic context, where the realities of practice have led to the use of pragmatic reasoning (Schell and Cervero, 1993).

These three different types of reasoning which OTs incorporate into their clinical reasoning are:

• theory-based reasoning;
• meaning-based reasoning;
• pragmatic reasoning.

These will be examined further and related to client-centred, social model thinking within housing. While it is acknowledged that the term 'clinical reasoning' is suggestive of the medical model, it will be used to maintain consistency with other literature.

Theory-based reasoning

This reasoning draws on theoretical knowledge to promote rational problem-solving. OTs within housing draw on a broad range of theory and knowledge, including OT, ergonomic, building, planning and biomedical theory as well as the socio-political approaches.

When planning intervention, OTs draw on an eclectic range of approaches developed across many disciplines. The rationale for much of OT intervention in housing remains based on biomedical and rehabilitation approaches (Munroe, 1996). An alternative approach has been based on the administrative process of matching clients to criteria for aids and adaptations, which has resulted in ambivalence about whether this constitutes 'proper OT' (Abraham and Clamp, 1991).

Craddock (1996a, b) suggests that the social model of disability was a more appropriate approach to use when problem-solving in housing. Its use is advocated for people with permanent impairments who are medically stable (Oliver, 1996); so it is clearly applicable for use with many people in the community setting and can be used alongside other approaches. Once the social model has been selected to inform practice, the focus of intervention becomes the removal of barriers, which include the built environment, attitudes and organisations. All three of these barriers will be considered further.

Built environment – the home

Barrier-free housing is fundamental to achieving equal rights in independent living (Hawkins and Stewart, 2002). Nowhere is the right for disabled people to participate fully in society more fundamental than within their own home. Despite this, there remains a shortage of accessible homes within the housing stock (Oliver and Barnes, 1998).

Over twenty years ago, Finlay (1978) introduced the idea of housing disability. This shifted the focus from performance capabilities of individuals, which she took as given, to restrictions imposed upon them by the structure of the house. The application of social model thinking would make it standard practice for OTs to be involved in the elimination of architectural barriers, especially in the home environment. This is not based on whether people fit set criterial; instead, it is based on their rights as citizens to participate equally in their community.

> We believe that it should not be regarded as an exotic idea for disabled children and those close to them to aspire to a quality of life comparable to that enjoyed by others . . . we start out by assuming that disabled children and their families should have access to experiences which others routinely expect, the issue then becomes one of finding the route to achieve it. (Read and Clements, 2001, pp. 14–15)

Overcoming the barrier of built environments is clearly an important role for OTs working in housing. This does not exclusively involve adapting properties, as this remains a segregated service which is in contrast to the social model's emphasis on integration into mainstream society based on participation, integration and equality (Priestley, 1999). Full integration necessitates the implementation of the principle of universal design to ensure that suitable housing is available as a mainstream provision (see Chapter 6).

While the focus of this book is on housing, broader changes in legislation have promoted accessibility to public buildings; so there are also opportunities for OTs to work to remove structural barriers in the wider community.

Attitudinal

A major attitudinal barrier faced by disabled people results from the power differential between themselves and professionals (Abberley, 1995; Oliver and Sapey, 1999). This affects who takes control over the decision-making process. Some clients continue to regard professionals as the authority figure and feel pressured to go along with recommendations they are not personally happy with (Stewart, 2000). Some professionals also hold a stereotyped view of disabled people, which expects them to behave as passive recipients of care to the extent that they are seen as aggressive if they take control of decisions affecting their own lives (French, 1994).

Case study 3.5: from author's practice
I visited a mother who had gained the reputation of being a 'difficult parent'. Her son had muscular dystrophy (MD), and they had recently moved into a wheelchair-accessible house. My first contact, which was to start considering additional adaptations, was a tense encounter. She had researched possible adaptations through the MD society, but previous experience had led her to expect a power struggle and that she would need to shout to make herself heard. Her immediate concern was the shower; so we focused on discussing her son's present and future needs, likes and dislikes in that area. We agreed to look through specific catalogues before the next visit. The breakthrough in the relationship came during the next meeting when we both opened the same catalogue, at the same page, and discovered that we had selected the same red adjustable shower seat. She realised that I had listened to her ideas, expected her to take an active part in the decision-making and that mutual decision-making was possible.

Research suggests that OT students have a tendency to focus on individualistic and personal tragedy approaches to disability, which could result in oppressive practice (Taylor, 1999). Craddock (1996a) observes that OTs, like other medical professions, remain unwilling to relinquish their right to assess and prescribe even when working with people in a stable condition when the intervention in question was a housing adaptation. It is acknowledged that professionals involved in arranging adaptations may actually be contributing to, rather than alleviating, disability (Hawkins and Stewart, 2002).

Medical model thinking can become an ingrained way of thinking which needs to be recognised and reconsidered (Heywood, 2001). An analysis of how a question is phrased can help identify whether someone was basing their view of disability on a medical or social model of disability (Oliver, 1990). This is a useful reflective tool to use in practice as the following questions demonstrate:

• I understand you are suffering from severe arthritis; does that make it difficult for you to get upstairs to your toilet?
• I noticed your only toilet is upstairs; does that cause you any problems?

It is also useful to examine the expectations of each party in the decision-making process. Craddock (1996b) argues that this barrier of professional attitudes could be overcome by a greater adoption of the social model, which would include relinquishing the authority gained through association with medicine.

Organisational

Organisational barriers are encountered by disabled people when they attempt to access adaptations or transfer to more appropriate housing. Poor publicity of the availability of grants creates an initial barrier for potential service users (Awang, 2002), as can the lack of direct contact with an OT adviser. The adaptation system itself is a complicated bureaucratic one for clients to navigate (Adams, 1996). Long waiting times for assessment and subsequent adaptation work along with unrealistic means tests to restrict the number of people receiving the housing services they need (Heywood, 1994). Disabled people are also insufficiently involved in decision-making, and information and advice on available housing options are often limited (Nocon and Pleace, 1997).

OTs can find themselves involved in administering organisational systems, which can appear designed to keep departments running rather than address the needs of clients (Hawkins and Stewart, 2002). This can result in a fundamental conflict of loyalties as they attempt to balance the twin requirements of empowering service users and acting as agents for the organisation (Abraham and Clamp, 1991). While effective management should take responsibility for strategic planning, managing staffing and financial resources, the experience of OTs can be that their attention is often diverted away from the focus of their job towards managerial issues.

Recognising these organisational barriers and having a clear understanding of the social model perspective can help OTs make conscious decisions about how to practise in this challenging situation. The promotion of the OT role as a consultant to keep disabled people fully informed and to help them navigate the complex housing systems becomes a priority. Examples of good practice include telephone advice services and service-user-led partnerships with OT services operating from resources centres to provide advice and information for potential users of the DFG system. It is necessary to identify organisational barriers and work to overcome them.

Case study 3.6: from author's practice

I returned from holiday to find that one of my clients (who had severe RA) and her husband had accepted a transfer to a council property. They had visited the house, but as the security shutters were up she had been unable to step over these to enter the house. The electricity had been disconnected so they were unable to try the stairlift. When I visited them a week later, she was going upstairs by standing on the footrest and leaning over the seat of the stairlift. The curved stairs were too narrow for her to go up seated with the limited flexion she had in her knees. The organisational system had pressured them into making a rushed decision with insufficient information.

Application of the social model theory to problem-solving in housing challenges OTs to work with disabled people, to focus on removing their barriers rather than becoming a disabling barrier themselves.

Meaning-based reasoning

Clinical reasoning within OT does not just involve the application of theory to practice; the uniqueness of individuals also needs to be considered (Mattingly, 1991a). Meaning-based reasoning is concerned with the subjective human world of motive, value and belief, which must to be taken into account in order to individualise interventions. This way of thinking recognises that there are no absolute right or wrong answers when planning intervention, instead it aims to decide what is best for a given client at a specific moment in time. This approach is necessary when collaborating to plan interventions which will be meaningful to clients (Mattingly and Fleming, 1994). It underpins client-centred practice and is an essential ingredient in the clinical reasoning of every OT.

While models of disability can aid understanding at a theoretical level, disability is actually experienced differently by every individual. Disabled people and their families are the experts on the lived realities of the problems they encounter. The refusal to listen to and consult with them has been justifiably described as professional arrogance (Davis, 1993). There is, therefore, a clear need to understand the client's perspective as part of the problem-solving process. This includes an understanding of their meaning of home and of family roles and dynamics and is an essential component to client-centred decision-making.

Understanding the meaning of home

> A house is more than four walls which hold up a roof and enclose a variety of functional spaces. For all of us, it is the basis of our security and our exploration of the world. It is the place where we find our privacy, express our personality and preferences and experiment with change. (Shearer, 1981, p. 125)

In the process of adapting houses, the meaning of home can be overlooked (Hawkins and Stewart, 2002). The home environment is often assumed to be flexible enough to accommodate adaptations, but this fails to acknowledge its psychological significance. Hasselkus (2002) states that the consideration of this sense of meaning would shift our attention from space to place.

Case study 3.7: from author's practice
The importance of understanding the subjective meaning of home to individuals was reinforced for me while interviewing two men after

adaptation work had been completed to their respective homes for a research project (Heywood, 2001).

There were many observable similarities between the two men. They were both in their seventies, living with their wives in ex-council houses which they had purchased under the right-to-buy scheme. Their houses had a similar layout with the stairs clearly visible from the front door. They also had a similar level of functional ability and both experienced severe difficulty climbing stairs.

The first man described his stairlift as 'the best thing since sliced bread'.

The second had declined to consider a stairlift as part of his adaptation work on the basis that 'it would have taken away my last remaining shred of dignity'.

Clinical reasoning in housing clearly needs to take account of the fact that a home is not just a physical environment but also a place of social and emotional significance. Client choice is therefore essential. This includes choice in the aesthetic appearance of an adaptation, as research has shown that adaptations can be rejected for this reason (Nocon and Pleace, 1997). This type of reasoning requires innovative and creative thinking, which need not have major cost implications. As one mother commented to the author on a follow-up visit:

> I was afraid that the shower room would feel clinical, but simply adding the frog tiles has transformed it into a fun room we can enjoy.

Understanding the importance of family roles and dynamics

Other significant areas to consider from the client's perspective are the roles and dynamics within the family or whatever social context in which they are living. When reflecting on adaptation work with a family which included a child with a degenerative disease, Medhurst and Ryan (1996a, b) recognised that the OT needed to reach deep into the personal territory of the family. Each family is unique with its own story to tell, and narrative reasoning (Mattingly, 1991b) was shown to be an effective way to allow the OT to place their expertise within the life context of the family and to understand the potential impact of adaptations on that family. Within this case study, the mother expressed her desire to have her child sleeping nearby, revealing her expectations of herself as his mother. This enabled the OT to realise that downstairs facilities were not an option this family would consider at this time. While recognising the potentially controversial nature of their claim, it was suggested that permanent solutions to family housing problems were unlikely. This was not due to any failure on the part of the OT to find the 'right adaptation' but recognised that meaning-based reasoning involved understanding the changing nature of family life. This requires OTs to focus on the best solution for a family at a particular point in time.

Client-centred decision-making

Mutual decision-making depends on mutual understanding which requires skills in listening, explaining and negotiating (Higgs and Jones, 2000). Meaning-based reasoning encourages the OT to understand the significance of disability, home and family from the perspective of each individual client. Having focused on listening to the client, they are then in a position to discuss the range of options and resources available to them. This type of client-centred decision-making is based on an understanding of the OT role as being a resource to enable clients to make informed decisions, rather than themselves being expert decision-makers. Without adequate consultation, there is the risk of providing adaptations which are seen as a violation to the home and which reinforce dependency; with it they can enhance the home and improve self-respect, dignity and self-worth (Heywood, 2001).

Pragmatic reasoning

This third type of reasoning moves beyond understanding the client to the practical reality of service delivery (Schell, 1998). It recognises that the context in which clinical reasoning occurs impacts upon the decisions which are made. It considers what is possible within the given circumstances of local resources and policy and national legislation. If therapists view themselves as autonomous professionals and only reason in accordance with their theoretical perspectives and values, they would fail to recognise the impact of their own environmental context (Chapparo and Ranka, 2000). From the critical perspective:

> Economic structures determine the roles of professionals as gate-keepers of scarce resources, legal structures determine their controlling functions as administrators of services. (Oliver, 1993, p. 54)

Every OT who has worked in local authorities will recognise the significance of contextual issues and the impact they have on practice. Government funding is limited and efficient, accountable use of resources is promoted at local levels. Increasing referral rates resulting in waiting lists, limited budgets and staff shortages are all familiar issues which are encountered regularly in this setting. All decisions regarding housing adaptations, or moving to a more suitable property, are taken within the context of current legislation as well as local criteria and resources. Research confirmed that pragmatic reasoning has a strong influence on the thinking and decision-making of OTs in housing (Munroe, 1996). An example given related to the local policy of initially providing only basic bathing equipment. OTs adhered to this policy despite their own judgement that the equipment would often be of limited benefit to the client and would delay the request for more appropriate equipment or adaptations. Specifications for larger adaptations can also be affected by grant limits and a lack of top-up money (Heywood, 2001). These are just two examples of pragmatic decision-taking and the dilemmas OTs face when there is conflict between what therapists perceive should be done, what the client wants to be done and what the system will allow (Chapparo and Ranka, 2000).

Pragmatic reasoning can place pressure on OTs to move away from client-centred, social model thinking. The combination of a high demand for OT involvement and limited resources can result in screening and prioritising systems which stem from an administrative model of disability. The persistence of medical model thinking within OT decision-making has been seen as a coping mechanism to deal with the existing shortage of resources (Heywood, 2001). There are two options for OTs seeking to work in partnership with disabled people in these circumstances – to operate as effectively as possible within the existing system or to challenge the system itself.

Work effectively within the system

Mattingly and Gilette (1991) argue that clinical reasoning and reflection could help devise more individualised strategies for clients even within rigid systems. They observe that experienced clinicians are better able to bend the rules of the system and that explicit clinical reasoning enhances their ability to put a case across to influential colleagues and budget holders.

To work effectively and argue their case within the system, OTs need a good, up-to-date knowledge of that system, including legislation, guidance and precedents set by case law as well as a recognition that local criteria exist as flexible guidelines to practise rather than absolute rules. While legislation does not protect OT practice against lack of resources, it can be empowering as it imposes duties upon local authorities which they are required to carry out, as well as providing powers which they are able to undertake. However, research suggests that OTs may not always make full use of the mandatory provision opportunities for DFGs (Heywood, 2001). These included omitting bathing (for which no medical need is required under the legislation), heating, caring for someone else, access to kitchen, items related to sensory impairment and access to a garden. The Human Rights Act 1998 can also serve as a statutory reinforcer of good practice and it will remain necessary to keep up to date with developments, including how articles are interpreted: including article 3 (which relates to torture – clients should not be forced to accept equipment or adaptations they do not want), and article 8 (which relates to rights surrounding private and family life and the home) (Clements and Read, 2003). It provides an opportunity for OTs to work with disabled people to present the case for more accessible housing.

In this situation of statutory obligations existing alongside limited resources, best practice requires that OTs ensure clients' legal rights are upheld while spending resources wisely on adaptations which will be effective for clients and their families. Research has shown that the grant limit, which was designed to save money, has actually led to wasted spending as insufficient space or limited heating can restrict the usefulness of adaptations (Heywood, 2001). Examples from this research include a couple who could not use their ground-floor-bedroom extension in the winter because it was too cold to sleep in and a woman who struggled to use her shower safely because it was not big enough to allow her to sit down. While working within the existing system, the effectiveness of adaptations can be maximised through consultation, attention to detail, the checking of work in progress to ensure there is no deviation from agreed plans, which would have a negative impact on outcomes, and preventing waste on unacceptable or inadequate adaptations (Heywood, 2001).

Challenge the system

The second option available to OTs is to work alongside disabled people to challenge the system and thereby alter the context in which they work. Political action, aimed at changing policy to promote the rights of disabled people, is the major focus of the disability rights movement. The social model perspective places broad responsibilities upon therapists working with individual clients. It is increasingly accepted that professionals have a broader role – to work alongside disabled people in shaping policy changes (Hawkins and Stewart, 2002).

If national legislation and funding arrangements or local policies are preventing people with disabilities from accessing suitable housing, then OTs have a role to play. This can be done at national and local levels, to promote the rights of disabled people within mainstream housing provision or through involvement in campaigns to increase funding levels, change means-testing procedures for DFGs and broaden provision available under mandatory grants. A recent example is the Home Fit for Children campaign, stemming from an investigation into DFG provision for families with disabled children (Beresford and Oldham, 2000). A coalition of parents and professionals formed to fight for the abolition of the means test on parents, and OTs were involved in providing evidence of the negative impact of the means test on families.

While planning intervention in housing, OTs need to balance these three types of reasoning, to ensure they are rational, appropriate to the individual and realistic in the circumstances. A clear focus on socio-political approaches and client-centredness can help overcome the opposing tendency to become an administrator within the housing system.

Conclusion

This chapter has explored clinical reasoning and the impact of the social model on that process within housing. It has considered the distinct ways in which the medical and social models of disability impact on how a problem is initially understood and how this influences the subsequent goals of intervention. The importance of the social model was recognised with the caveat that this should be used within the holistic and client-centred framework embodied in OT models of practice.

Further investigation into the wider implications of the medicalisation of disability and socio-political approaches was applied to the shift in power relationships between professionals and disabled people. Decision-making in housing should be made in collaboration with disabled people, not based on the idea that professionals know best.

The complexity of problem-solving and decision-making in housing was recognised, and linked to the importance of OTs becoming more aware of their clinical reasoning. Three different types of reasoning used by OTs in practice were identified. It was suggested that these could be used as a framework for reflective practice to ensure client-centred, social model intervention in housing. The use of social model ideas in theory-based reasoning will ensure that OTs work to overcome architectural, attitudinal and organisational barriers which restrict people's opportunities to participate equally in society. Meaning-based reasoning can ensure that practice remains client-centred by understanding what disability, home and family mean to individual clients. Pragmatic reasoning can ensure that OTs work effectively within the existing system and also challenge that system to help promote the rights of disabled people.

Key points

- Decisions relating to housing intervention have major long-term effects on people's homes. These decisions need to be made in partnership with disabled people and based on sound clinical reasoning.
- A deeper understanding of the social model and clinical reasoning can enhance an OT's decision-making within housing through the use of

reflective practice. It can also lead to the development of a firm evidence base within this setting.

- Socio-political approaches have the potential to transform relationships between professionals and disabled people by moving away from treating people like patients in hospital towards working with citizens in the community.
- OTs in housing should adopt a consultative role, focusing on the identification and removal of barriers in partnership with disabled people. They are challenged to focus on removing barriers without becoming barriers themselves.
- When working closely with people's homes and families, meaning-based reasoning is essential to provide interventions acceptable to the individual.
- Full knowledge of legislation, ongoing consultation and attention to detail can help OTs work effectively within the system. The responsibilities of OTs in housing include challenging the system itself.

CHAPTER 4

Housing: the user's perspective

SALLY FRENCH AND JOHN SWAIN

This chapter considers housing from the viewpoint of disabled people in Britain. It is based upon interviews and writings by disabled people who have substantial experience of housing issues and considerable contact with occupational therapists. The main message of this chapter is that choice and control by disabled people is central to the satisfactory outcome of securing a suitable home. It is also clear that accessible housing is of limited use unless the wider environment is also accessible.

Moving to independent living in the community

Until relatively recent times, large numbers of disabled adults were compelled to live either with their parents or within institutions, but with the rise of the disabled people's movement in the 1970s this situation started to change. Disabled people who lived in institutions devised imaginative schemes (which were usually opposed by professionals) in order to live within the community and to gain some control of their lives. An early initiative was the Grove Road scheme, where residents of an institution negotiated with a housing association to build a block of flats for disabled and non-disabled tenants. The non-disabled tenants paid a subsidised rent in exchange for offering their services to the disabled tenants (Davis, 1981). Oliver and Barnes state that:

> the principal objective behind the scheme was that it should not be conspicuous, but must blend into the local community and must cater for disabled people's needs in the privacy of their own homes in a way that encourages and supports independence and individuality. (1996, p. 82)

At the same time, the residents of a Cheshire Home, Le Court in Hampshire, persuaded the local authority to enable them to live in the community. It was not only suitable housing that was required but also the provision of personal assistants. Briggs (1993) gives a graphic account of the struggles she experienced in reaching her goal of community living:

> I hadn't anticipated so much pressure in my new life. I had not been prepared for the volume of decisions I had to make. Simple things, such as sorting out looing routines; how to use the local laundrette; finding out where all the allowances come from and how to get them; sorting out local tradespeople; sorting out dustbin collections, milk deliveries, a doctor, a chemist, and so on. But the worst thing was the incomplete building work, I was trying to start a new life on a building site . . . Sometimes I thought that within a few months I would be back in Le Court, because I did not think that I could continue. (1993, p. 134)

These early initiatives, which involved enormous energy and struggle on the part of disabled people, have, over time, led to legislation, such as the Direct Payments Act 1996, whereby local authorities grant disabled people a sum of money, following an assessment, to buy their own personal care. The Disability Discrimination Act 1995 also requires modifications to be made to buildings 'where reasonable'. This legislation is weak, however, and 'less favourable treatment' can still be justified on a variety of grounds, including those of health and safety (Hogan, 2001).

Despite some advances, it is still the case that many disabled people live in unsuitable housing, including institutions, and that many, too, have been unable to leave their childhood homes. Morris (1990) believes that disabled people who live in institutions should be considered homeless as homelessness does not necessarily imply living on the street but includes living in unsatisfactory conditions such as in hostels and bed and breakfast accommodation (Pryke, 1998). Esther Hurdle, a disabled woman with four children, for instance, lived in a hospital ward for three years while adaptations were being made to her home (Peace, 2003). What then are the housing options for disabled people, the barriers to and opportunities for independent living in the community?

Housing options for disabled people

Barriers to independent living in the community

Disabled people are among the poorest in the country and are less likely than others to own their own homes (Burns, 2000). However, even if disabled people are homeowners, they may be disadvantaged:

> Housing departments often exclude homeowners from being eligible for rehousing. The property of disabled owner-occupiers may be totally unsuitable for them. They may consequently be unable to leave hospital or

institutional care, may be made dependent on others or imprisoned within a physically unsuitable home. (Morris, 1993, p. 139)

Money for maintenance and repair may also be limited (Peace, 2003), and disabled people are often 'stuck' in their homes with little prospect of moving or, alternatively, having to move when they want to stay. Rabiee et al. (2001) highlight the lack of choice available to disabled young people, especially those with learning difficulties, who may be denied housing opportunities because of a lack of appropriate support. Hawker and King (1999) found that only 7 per cent of people with learning difficulties owned their own home or had a private tenancy, 53 per cent lived with their parents and the remainder lived in various types of residential settings.

Marginalised groups, including many disabled people, occupy the worst housing, and this impacts particularly on disabled women (Morris, 1993) and black disabled people (Drake, 1996). As Abberley states:

The least satisfactory housing tends . . . to be that inhabited by sections of the population of which disabled people form a disproportionately large percentage: elderly people and people on low incomes. (1993, p. 113)

Beresford and Oldham (2002) interviewed the parents of disabled children regarding their housing. Nine out of ten families reported at least one problem, with the most common being a lack of space. A third found the location of their home unsuitable and only a minority had received statutory assistance. White families were more likely to be suitably housed than black families. Bevan (2002) found that families appreciated information and being treated as individuals (rather than being fitted into an existing framework). They were appreciative if the needs of children, for example opportunities for play, were considered.

It has been known since Victorian times that the quality of housing impacts on people's physical and mental health (Best, 1997). This is no less true today, although it is difficult to disentangle the effects of housing from other factors such as low income, especially when the worst housing problems have been solved. Housing has been central to social policy for the past hundred years (Baldock et al., 1999) from the building of 'garden cities' (such as Welwyn Garden City) and new towns (such as Stevenage and Bracknell) to the building of tower blocks and council estates. The effect of such projects on people's health and well-being has ranged from beneficial to disastrous but has always largely excluded the needs of disabled people.

The housing options for disabled people, then, are determined by the barriers they face in realising independent living in the community and all the broader consequences for quality of life. Within this analysis are factors that are beyond the scope of this chapter to examine in detail. These factors are generated by the diversity of disabled people which reflects the diversity of the general population in Britain and includes income, age differences and the diverse needs of ethnic minority communities. When considering the needs of disabled people worldwide, diversity is even greater although disabled people have found, through organisations such as Disabled People's International, that there is also much commonality in their experiences and aspirations (Stone, 1999).

'Special needs housing': overcoming barriers?

One policy aimed at overcoming such barriers to independent living in the community has been the development of 'special needs housing'. In Britain there is a limited supply of special needs housing, most of which is owned by local authorities (Morris, 1990; Stewart et al., 1999). This consists of 'wheelchair accessible' housing and 'mobility' housing, which contain a few basic features such as a flat entrance into the house. The stock of special needs housing has always been inadequate and has declined since the 1970s despite the fact that it is cheaper to build accessible dwellings than to adapt inaccessible ones (Barnes et al., 1999). Between 1984 and 1989 local authorities and housing associations built 168,665 mainstream homes but only 1840 homes accessible to wheelchair users, while the private house-building sector built no wheelchair-accessible dwellings at all (Barnes, 1991). Resources for building public housing were drastically cut by the Conservative government of the 1980s, and the 'right to buy' policy meant that many council houses which would have been suitable for adaptation were sold. Between 1980 and 1988 homelessness among disabled people rose by 92 per cent and that did not include those who were living in institutions or with their parents (Oliver and Barnes, 1996). Johnstone (1998) states that there are over four million people in Britain with mobility impairments but only 80,000 accessible dwellings.

An irony is that a large proportion of wheelchair-accessible dwellings are occupied by people who do not use wheelchairs (Stewart, 2004). One of the reasons for this is that wheelchair-accessible housing usually provides single accommodation. Barnes and Mercer state:

> segregated 'special needs' housing remains central to government plans for 'community care'. Even so many of these properties do not satisfy people's requirements. For example too few have more than one bedroom, even though most disabled people live with families, and a significant minority of single disabled people need two bedroom housing to accommodate a personal assistant. (2003, pp. 50–1)

Stewart et al. interpret this situation in the following way:

> We argue that the individual model of disability led planners to regard disabled people as sexless and without families and that, as the

development of special housing was conceived as an alternative to residential care, the emphasis should be on the provision of one-person dwellings reflecting the single life style of many residents in these homes. (1999, p. 10)

Even if suitably sized housing is available, many dwellings are only partly adapted, and, if disabled people have savings, they may be compelled to spend them on house adaptations (Barnes et al., 1999). Many disabled people experience long delays in being assessed. Frazer and Glick quote one of their research participants as saying:

> When I moved into the area I was told there was an 18 month waiting list for an OT visit for assessment. I had to borrow money to pay for bathroom equipment and stair-lift as I could not wait 18 months as I have two small children to care for and I was not safe without this equipment. (2001, p. 21)

A further criticism of special needs housing is that it has concentrated almost exclusively on people with physical impairments rather than on other disabled people such as those with visual impairments (Imrie, 2004). Research undertaken by the Thomas Pocklington Trust (2003) found that, although the majority of older people who acquired a visual impairment did not alter their housing arrangements (partly because of its familiarity), others found changes to lighting and colour schemes useful and were concerned about the availability of natural light. They reported needing more space to house equipment and to work safely in the kitchen and preferred not to have to 'zig-zag' between rooms. Space was also important for entertaining friends especially as many people were unable to go out unaided. Some of the research participants spoke of problems with landlords when they required alterations to lighting or when they wanted white edges painted on communal stairs. Maintenance of the house and the upkeep of the garden also caused concern as did safety matters, such as climbing on chairs to reach high cupboards.

Beyond the issue of the limited supply of this type of housing, many disabled people reject the idea of 'special' housing, which has the potential to stigmatise and exclude, and would prefer housing to be designed with everybody's needs in mind. The full inclusion of disabled people requires that all housing is accessible. As Hurst states:

> Why do we have to move if we're disabled? Conversely why should we not be able to move once we have suitable accommodation? And why can't we visit our friends and neighbours? (1990, p. 9)

The concept of special needs housing has arisen through the medical model of disability where disabled people are viewed as different and abnormal. This policy is based on research into disablement that has focused on disabled people themselves, for example the number of people with particular impairments and the severity of those impairments, rather than investigating the physical and social environment. Oliver (1990, pp. 7–8) is critical of government surveys of disabled people (for example Martin et al., 1988) and has poignantly rephrased the questions (which are based on the medical model of disability) to questions that are underpinned by the social model. For example, instead of the question 'Can you tell me what is wrong with you?' he asks, 'Can you tell me what is wrong with society?' and instead of the question 'Did you move here because of your health problem/disability? he asks, 'What inadequacies in your housing caused you to move here?' Most research which has taken a social model approach has been undertaken by disabled people themselves (see Barnes and Mercer, 1997). Later in this chapter we review the implications of the social model for occupational therapists. Setting the scene generally, Macfarlane and Laurie state:

> This individual or 'medical' model has determined the range of services on offer to disabled people and how those services should be provided and has been the basis of the training for individuals working in the areas of health, rehabilitation, social work, residential, home care and 'special needs' housing. This training encourages professionals to pursue a role of influence in the lives of disabled people and to view themselves as experts on various aspects of disability. The experience and expertise of disabled people who face discrimination on a day-to-day basis is therefore seen as of little value. (1996, p. 7)

Towards accessible housing

The dissatisfaction with the very notion of special needs housing has led to the concept of 'Lifetime Homes' promoted by the Joseph Rowntree Foundation. Lifetime Homes are built with many standard features, such as a downstairs toilet and sufficient turning space for a wheelchair, and are built to be easily adjusted as circumstances change, allowing for, for example, the fitting of a stairlift (Macfarlane and Laurie, 1996). Stewart et al. state that:

> Lifetime houses can be thought of as universalist in that anyone could occupy them and in consequence they neither stigmatize nor create dependency, while the decision to adapt fully can still be related to individual needs and circumstances. (1999, p. 17)

The extension of the Building Regulations in 1999, whereby all newly built homes must meet certain criteria of accessibility, reflect this approach. Similar standards, such as switches and sockets at an appropriate height from the floor and a level approach to the principal entrance, have been produced by the Access Committee for England (Walker, 1995) and the Centre for Accessible Environments (Peace, 2003). These criteria do not, however, consider the needs of visually impaired people (Allen et al., 2002). In general terms, the identification of those characteristics in housing which make it usable or adaptable for people with a range of disabilities needs further investigation.

Other groups within society have also noted the inadequacy of housing design. Women, for example, have complained about the design of kitchens and the unsuitability of housing when caring for children (Peace, 2003). Imrie states:

> the myth of a 'normal' person, of the white male, has been a powerful dimension of the design process, yet one which has had and continues to have clear racist, sexist and ableist underpinnings. (1998, p. 133)

Part of the blame for this can be directed at architects who, according to Drake (1996), are often more concerned with aesthetics than function when designing buildings and expect people to perform in a uniform way. Imrie (1998) believes that disability, if considered at all, is usually an afterthought or is regarded as a 'special interest' in the curriculum of architects. This leads Walker to conclude that:

> to meet the challenges successfully architects must be prepared to learn from the people for whom they have been creating a disabling environment – the real experts who know about access needs. (1995, pp. 46–7)

Imrie asserts, however, that the work of architects must be put within a wider framework of social structures, values and ideologies and that architecture is 'pre-determined by political and economic power including laws, statuses, codes and corporate clients' (2004, p. 283).

Beyond accessible housing

It cannot be emphasised strongly enough that inclusion in society goes far beyond the design of domestic dwellings. The early pioneers of community living were well aware that accessible housing in isolation would not be sufficient. Personal assistance in the home may be required and, to become fully involved in the community, an accessible environment is essential in terms of accessible transport, public buildings and information, appropriate attitudes and behaviour, and flexible social structures which, for example, allow disabled people to participate in education and paid employment. Imrie states that:

> Western cities are characterized by a design apartheid where building form and design are inscribed into the values of an 'able-bodied' society . . . This has led some commentators to regard the built environment as disablist, that is projecting 'able-bodied' values which legitimate oppressive and

discriminatory practices against disabled people purely on the basis that they have physical and mental impairments. (1998, p. 129)

Allen et al. (2002) undertook research with visually impaired children concerning their housing needs. They, too, questioned presumptions about the significance of housing design:

children with visual impairment did not consider the built environment of the home and neighbourhood to be a problem. This is mainly because the visually impaired children were able to construct a memory map based on 'fixed' points (for example sounds, textures, objects and so on) in the built environment. These maps provided the visually impaired children with predictive confidence. (2002, p. 16)

This shows that people's own resources and coping strategies may be more efficient than adaptations and may render the need for adaptations unnecessary (Harrison, 2003). Allen et al. found, however, that the children needed a garden to increase their confidence and needed more space for equipment, which could be a problem if they shared a bedroom with a sibling. Minor adaptations to lighting were sometimes required. The outside environment could cause conflict between the visually impaired children and their parents because, whereas parents were inclined to respond to it by restricting the freedom of their children, the children themselves were prepared to develop strategies for coping with it and tended not to be intimidated. Older visually impaired people who acquire their impairments, however, are less inclined to venture out alone. In a survey by the RNIB (2002) 27 per cent of older visually impaired people did not feel confident enough to walk alone in their immediate neighbourhood.

Sue and Paul Nicholls, a blind couple interviewed by French et al. (1997), illustrate the contrast of functioning within the home and the outside environment. Paul said:

In your own home there is a more equal relationship because you can do things for other people . . . but when you're in a restaurant or pub you are reliant on other people. You've got to know a place very well before you can even get up and go to the toilet without asking for help. It's a very unequal situation indeed. (1997, p. 31)

Talking of bringing up their two sighted daughters, Sue said:

In a way it's an extension of your own life and your own home and that's where you feel capable and secure. We brought up the children as we wanted to, nobody interfered . . . Having the children wasn't a problem, it was under our control, and in our own environment; we were not being compared to what other people do either. Whatever we did it was normal to them. (1997, p. 32)

An understanding that the whole environment needs to be accessible has led to the concept of 'universal design', which has at its core the principle of designing for all people and in such a way that environments are flexible and adjustable. A major flaw, however, is that it ignores the political and social dimensions of inclusion. As Imrie (2004) points out:

> Its principles are apolitical in that there is little explicit recognition of the relationship between the social, technical, political and economic processes underpinning building and design. (2004, p. 282)

If disabled people are to be truly included in the community, then a profound transformation of society, in all its aspects, is required.

Disabled people's experiences of housing adaptations

This section of the chapter is based on interviews we conducted with disabled people who have had significant experiences with housing and who, between them, have experienced considerable contact with occupational therapists in recent times. Four interviews focus specifically on housing issues and were conducted for the specific purposes of this chapter; three others explore the relationship between occupational therapists and clients more generally. The purpose was not to provide a representative sample of service users but to gather some 'real world' experiences which we hope will illustrate some of the attributes clients value in therapists and some of the problems which may arise in occupational therapy from the client's viewpoint. The interviews also illustrate, with specific examples, many of the issues discussed above and found in disability studies literature.

Location

What, then, might be important to disabled people in relation to where they live? Perhaps not surprisingly, many issues were similar and, in a general sense, would be significant for many non-disabled people too. Location, for example, can matter for many different reasons.

David told us:

> Location, where it is, is very important to me. I like to have a degree of accessibility in and around where I live, so the site needs to be accessible, and then I would say that about quarter of a mile around would be nice to be accessible, though it's not top of my list because I have the car. So obviously proximate parking, or building adjacent covered parking, because to function, especially in the winter months, I need it to be right bang on my doorstep.

As a wheelchair user, access within the house starts for David with plenty of room to move around.

> Space, because I use the chair. Lots of space. I find that most adapted premises are short on space; unless they are purpose built for a wheelchair user, they are inadequate.

Access to the whole of the property, including the garden, is also important and, as David indicates, can have an impact on family life.

> One of the things that often falls short in terms of access for me is the garden. If it's there, I can't get to it. And I certainly think the way the grant schemes are structured at the moment that's a shortfall, particularly for things like child care – if you can't get to your garden, you can't supervise or care for your children adequately.

Dawn lives with her partner and seven children from previous marriages, two of whom are disabled. They have recently moved, and consideration of the whole family was crucial for Dawn. Access is clearly very significant, particularly as it provides a context for relationships within the family.

> It's important that the whole family have access around the entire house. That's the biggest priority. We have just moved house, and the thing that was imperative was that everyone could get access to every room, that includes the laundry room, the cupboards. Obviously for us having M with mobility difficulties, and balance, it means that there has got to be circulation space . . . It's single storey. The reason for that is simply that M has access without having to shout for anybody. It is terribly intrusive to have to ask somebody to escort you if you feel you would like to go on your own, and M does like to wander round on his own.

Home is where the heart is

A major theme in the interviews was that a house is not simply a place to live but a 'home' with all the psychological and social connotations this holds. Housing issues for disabled people, as for non-disabled people, are certainly more than the building or place. Home can play a part in making manifest a personal identity. Having a home, and having the choice to stay within it, is of the utmost importance to most people. Norman (1998), talking of older people, states:

> It is not sufficiently realised that the loss of one's home – however good the reasons for losing it – can be experienced as a form of bereavement and can produce the same grief reaction as the loss of a close relative. (1998, p. 76)

Even if the home is not entirely suitable physically, many people still prefer to stay where they are because of the memories and associations that surround it (Peace, 2003).

Case study 4.1

Barbara is a woman losing her sight in old age. The notion of home, together with associated relationships, is clearly apparent in the following exchange:

Sally	Have you made any changes to your house since you had problems with your sight?
Barbara	No. I haven't made any changes at all because I've lived here so long I know the number of stairs to go up and down. The two steps we have in the passage don't bother me because I know where they are. It might be a different problem if I was moving to a new place to live.
Sally	Would it put you off moving?
Barbara	I wouldn't want to move from here, because I like the house and we've got it nice and warm and it's convenient – not too far from the shops. Crossing the road is a difficulty, but I'm fortunate that I have a husband who always accompanies me, but it must be very, very difficult for somebody on their own.

The notion of home is linked with many personal and social understandings, including comfort, security, love, caring, quality of life and lifestyle – although it can, of course, be associated with the lack of these qualities. Central to this is choice and control – or lack of choice and control. Home is the place that we make our own, the expression of ourselves, starting with the choice of where we live. Choice is, of course, always limited, and disability can play a major part in such limitations.

Choice is important for Arlene, a woman with multiple impairments and a powerchair user, but her experience illustrates what it is like to have no choice:

I had no choice in the area where I had to live when I became disabled. It was a choice of living here or living in hospital. This house was found for me and adapted while I spent a year in hospital. I hadn't been in this area before, and I didn't know anybody. So not only was I facing the fact that I was going to be disabled, and that was a new experience, I had no social network round here. I came into sort of an alien environment; they didn't want a disabled resident to live here and I wasn't told this. I have approached counsellors and said, 'Get me out of here' on numerous occasions, and they've said, 'Well, we can put you in a pensioner's bungalow but it is too small for your needs' . . . The housing situation is also that I've got such an array of adaptations now that to re-house me would cost them a lot of money and they are not prepared to do that.

The limitation of choice experienced by Arlene is not restricted to bricks and mortar.

They actually got a petition up to stop a disabled person moving in here. So I came in, said hello to my neighbours and was told we don't want you . . . like you shouldn't be in the building: you should be in an institution. They [professionals] put me in a situation where I faced harassment. They hadn't explored the environment I was going to be living in. They also caused problems because they asked able-bodied people where my ramp should be situated, rather than asking me, and even to this day, it's 13 years since I moved here, my ramp is at the back of the building and the able-bodied people come in at the front. Up 'til about two years ago, I had no lighting coming in at the rear entrance because it's down past garages. They didn't have a street light there so it was jet black . . . The tenants, even after 13 years, have caused problems . . . I had to seek advice from a solicitor. I got a warning letter about my conduct as a tenant from the council saying that I was slamming doors within the flat, and it's an open-plan flat – there's only one sliding door and the other one's automatic. So they hadn't checked anything out. They complained about my district nurses coming in in the morning, they come in at 8.30, and they complained about the noise the nurses made coming into the building. So the council, instead of telling them to get lost, carpeted the outside of the flat – it's the only block of flats here to have any carpeting – and there was also in the letter of complaint about the fact that my wheelchair left trailing marks, as I came in the back door, on the carpet.

Experiences with occupational therapists

Turning to experiences with occupational therapists, the theme of choice and control, or lack of it, again ran through this strand of the interviews. This was apparent in both positive and negative examples. When communication breaks down, or is never initiated in an equal manner, the possibility of choice and control by the person involved is precluded, or contested.

The power relationship with the occupational therapist and Kate's resistance to it is clearly apparent in the language that she uses to describe her experiences with occupational therapists, such as 'battle'.

What I did find incredibly difficult to come to terms with was somebody coming into my home and saying, 'This needs to be done and this is how it's gong to be done.' I had no say whatsoever to the point where . . . well one of the things is the front door which is completely flat because I'm in a wheelchair. I could cope with a small rise very easily and I demonstrated that I could manage. What happens now is that whenever you open the door the leaves blow in because it's so flat. I had quite a long argument, added to which the builder had difficulty finding such a flat front door.

The other thing is the front lounge: it was designed without any discussion. I couldn't deviate from it one millimetre. It was designed as an adaptation without any thought to the fact that it was affecting my home and that it wasn't just me that it affected.

The only battle that I won, and it was a major argument that held up all the work for about three months, was that they wanted to lower all the worktops in the kitchen to my height and I kept pointing out that there were three other members of the family and I didn't want to have to do all the work! What we actually did was a carpenter friend of mine put rollout tops under the existing tops so I have something my height and they've got something at their height. It was as if I was living on my own and that the property was theirs.

The other major argument I had was that initially they weren't going to put a stairlift in at all [Kate has a ground floor and a basement]. They said I could live on the top level. I pointed out that I had two teenage daughters who would be completely cut off from me and I wanted to know what was going on down there. It was partly expense, but they weren't looking at me holistically at all. I did get the stairlift but it wasn't done in the first wave; it was an ongoing argument. She just came in, there was no awareness of me as a person, it was a practical issue – we had to get a wheelchair around this building. But I'm a person – it's not a wheelchair that has to go through that door, it's me!

Harrison (2003) warns that:

Although it is useful to highlight particular physical environmental barriers and possibilities for improvement, this should not lead to disaggregating aspects of environment in a formulaic way that suits the divisions of professional expertise, or follows the demarcation of academic preoccupations and disciplines. (2003, p. 10)

A similar experience to Kate's is apparent in Arlene's narrative. Here she describes her first involvement in occupational therapy and the agendas and values that she confronted.

My first experience was after I was given the wheelchair in hospital when I was in for that year. I was in the middle of doing my OU degree and studied from my bed because I was in my bed more often when I was in hospital. I got pushed, because I didn't have my powerchair, to the occupational therapy department one day and they said to me did I want to make a cake or make a basket and I didn't want to do either. I said, 'What else?' and she said, 'No, you can either make a cake or make a basket or you can fry an egg'; that was the other thing they suggested. And I thought, 'Well, this is great. I have no interest in doing this' and I would rather be doing what I was doing in the first place, which was reading my book. They didn't think I had any need to do any sort of study. As a disabled person I wasn't going

to be able to cope with cooking and things within my home environment –
I probably wouldn't have baked a cake if I hadn't been disabled and I wasn't
going to start just because they wanted me to.

In her interview, Arlene provided a number of examples where she experienced considerable difficulty in having her views heard or believed. For
instance, she had been experiencing difficulties closing the back door to
her block of flats and the other tenants started to complain that the door
was being left open.

> So I started to get notices pinned on the back door that said, 'Please keep this
> door locked at all times, close the door.' And if I put two wheels over my ramp
> they would slam the door even if I was going into my garden area and I've
> always had to have keys to get back in. An OT visited me . . . and I explained
> that I couldn't drive the wheelchair and shut the door, and she said could
> they attach a hook thing onto my shoulder that would hook on the door and,
> if I was able to manoeuvre the chair properly, this hook would grab onto this
> other thing and the door would shut behind me. And I thought, 'Well, I might
> get decapitated or something.' I said, 'I don't think that's going to work.' It
> took many, many months for the OT system to put this right. I had to
> demonstrate that I couldn't actually shut the door to three different people . . .
> then they said, yes, I could have my remote on that door.

Dawn had similar experiences. From her viewpoint, occupational therapists are limited in what they can do by the system.

> I think the difficulties have been with the previous OT. She was all too aware
> of what she was allowed to recommend from a financial point of view and
> she was very aware of what the process was . . . But instead of saying . . .
> 'We aren't going to get funding for a downstairs toilet until M is eight
> because that's the way the system works', if she'd said, 'Yes, I really feel that
> M is entitled to a downstairs toilet, of course he should have a toilet, but I
> just cannot get it for him', then I could have understood that. But she
> didn't; she kept saying that until he's eight he doesn't need a toilet
> downstairs. And she'd turn up with commodes and all sorts of ridiculous
> equipment.

A power relationship between therapist and client has many elements,
including the provision of house designs and equipment determined by
the therapist and the style of relationship initiated by the therapist. Sandy,
for instance, found her occupational therapist distant and inflexible and
was helped by a friend and her carer when the equipment from the occupational therapist could not be used:

> When I got home, the social service OT came and she started as if it was day
> one with a big assessment when I'd had the whole thing done in hospital.
> I was ill and in a lot of pain, sick most of the time, couldn't eat, and I

couldn't be doing with it. I thought, 'Just go away – just go to the hospital and they'll tell you everything you want to know.' She was neutral. She was just doing her job with her clipboard. I can't remember her name – she was just a professional. She came back to say that there was a waiting list for this bath thing so I'd have to have bed baths for three months from the carer. Finally, this thing arrived. None of us knew it was coming. It came with a man in a van – a lovely, friendly man with this contraption – but it didn't fit. We got to 'breaking rule time' then which meant 'blow what they said'. My friend and my carer got these two boards and they made a slide system to the bath. The OT didn't help one bit. When we told her the contraption wouldn't work, she said, 'Well, that's that then: it will have to be bed baths.' She never came again.

Kevin objects to going through occupational therapists for the equipment he needs:

If you want a spade to dig your garden, you don't go to an OT, do you? You go down the hardware shop and buy a spade, the one that suits you. So why can't I go down to my local hardware shop and buy a buttonhook, or buy a stick, or buy anything? A tool is a tool.

For assistance to be given with housing issues, the organisation and the professional must first recognise that these issues need addressing. In Barbara's case, her needs were not recognised, and this lack of recognition may reflect both her age and her impairment:

I never had advice. The only thing that I was asked was if I had a magnifying glass. Well, there are hundreds of different types but you have to find out for yourself what suits you. I was a bit disillusioned when all they said was, 'Have you got a magnifying glass?' It's not very substantial, is it?

We will end this section with some advice from disabled people. This begins with some good experiences with occupational therapists. When there is choice and control on the part of the home user and a true working partnership with the occupational therapist, creative and satisfactory ideas emerge giving a very positive experience. For Dawn and David this was when occupational therapists recognised their agendas and took their side.

Dawn thinks the occupational therapist who is working with her son at present is constrained by finance, but, nevertheless, she backs Dawn rather than the system.

She makes recommendations that are clearly based on what she believes to be right, and she listens and [is] prepared to alter according to family circumstances. An example of that would be when she originally looked at our old house for rails around the house, she made the recommendation, came back for comments and took on board what I had to say, and made some alterations. She's also got off the fence and written to local authorities, complained and pleaded with them to alter kerbs, pavements, roads around the house. It is not part of her brief really, but she is prepared to do that.

David has had similar experiences of occupational therapists joining forces with him.

> When I was being offered accommodation by the local authority and the housing association, it was very useful to have the OT there who could say, 'Well no, that's not actually suitable for this person.' That I found useful because I felt very pressured to just take somewhere to live whenever I was offered somewhere. I was in crisis, and I was thinking, 'No, this isn't right; this will not work', and I was really worried that I wouldn't be able to get out . . . I found that they reassured me and fought my corner, which was to say, 'Don't you worry: stop in that short-term accommodation as long as you need to, until it's right for you. Don't feel pressured to take something that's 75 per cent of the way towards something you are after if you physically can't cope with it' . . . So I think they give you psychological support as well because of their expertise when everyone else was saying, 'Well, it's a disabled flat so just get yourself in there.'

Arlene and Dawn offer advice to occupational therapists which emanates from the central theme of choice and control and emphasises the need for active listening. The first quotation is from Arlene, who puts a particular emphasis on the need to recognise that it is the client's home environment. Dawn then underlines the importance of recognising the particular values adhered to by the family.

> Remember that the person you are going in to, it's their home environment and it's never an extension of the hospital ward. You are not in control. You have got to respect the person that you are going in to. Treat them with dignity and listen to what they say because the disabled person is living the disability and they are the experts.

> To listen. To do as much listening and understanding as possible. Not to take your own agendas into your workplace, and your own personal experiences. We all have a perception of what is a good family life, what constitutes acceptable levels of access, but just because an OT feels that they know what's right for a client, doesn't mean it's going to work . . . Even the ones that have good practice, there's still the underlying attitude that the best thing for the child is to be independent, and it comes down to what independence is all about. Independence for my child, as far as I am concerned, is not being able to walk up and down stairs by himself. Independence is choosing whether or not he ever wants to go up the stairs again. It is not about getting the best out of somebody physically. I am not aiming to produce an Olympic champion; I want a content, well-rounded child.

Conclusion

Esmond et al. (1998) undertook a three-year research project which kept the views of disabled people at its centre, as in the present chapter. They conclude that housing could not be examined in isolation as it is linked to appropriate assistance and access to all community facilities. They provide a range of principles that can be applied regardless of the particular housing scheme adopted and an appropriate conclusion to the discussions in this chapter.

The principles include:

- an understanding of what independent living means in practice;
- participation and control by disabled people;
- access to independent advocacy support;
- security of tenure;
- financial control over services if that is what disabled people want;
- size of housing scheme appropriate to the tenants' choice, control, independence and privacy;
- accessibility of the local and wider community;
- good liaison among agencies – housing departments, social services, health authorities and disabled people's groups;
- flexibility and a range of housing to take account of disability and change;
- accessible and adaptable housing;
- promotion of disability equality at all levels of organisations;
- sensitivity to the needs of people from ethnic minorities;
- housing which is integrated into the community rather than being grouped together as special needs housing;
- flexible support which is not tied to any one building.

They conclude that:

> disabled people want the same as non-disabled people, the opportunity to live in their own homes, with whom they choose or by themselves, to participate in their local communities and to have a reasonable quality of life. (Esmond et al., 1998, p. 31)

Imrie goes further when he states:

> One of the most significant problems for disabled people relates to physical obstacles and barriers within the built environment. Many commercial and public buildings are inaccessible to wheelchair users, while few buildings provide appropriate design features to enable people with a range of sensory impairments to move around with confidence and ease. Accessible public transport is a rarity while most housing lacks basic adaptations or design features to facilitate independent living for disabled people . . . As

> some have argued this is tantamount to an infringement of disabled people's civil liberties. (2004, p. 279)

Macfarlane and Laurie (1996) provide a long list of recommendations which include the need for professionals to acquire a full understanding of the social model of disability, the need for organisations of disabled people to be adequately funded to enable their full involvement in planning and consultation and a move away from the notion that disabled people have 'special' housing needs. Gans (1968) makes the important point that the design of any building or environment does not necessarily determine how it will be used. This will depend on the social system and culture of those who inhabit it. In support of this argument Harrison (2003) states:

> it would be unfortunate if design, housing planning practitioners and researchers were to focus on classifications, categorisations, measurement, design methods and technological advances without a full regard to the ways in which physical features are actually 'received' by housing consumers. (2003, p. 10)

It is clear that thorough consultation with disabled people is essential but, until there is sufficient political will to make society inclusive to all disabled people, it is naive to imagine that accessible private dwellings will be anything more than a nominal gesture. Similarly, if the impact of occupational therapists is to move beyond tokenism, they need to heighten their awareness of disability from the perspective of disabled people, work in partnership with disabled people to remove disabling barriers, recognise the expertise of disabled people and use their professional power to assist disabled people in their struggle for full participative citizenship.

Key points

From the literature and the illustrations in this chapter, there are various principles which can be applied across housing work with disabled people:

• Occupational therapists need a very sound understanding of disability and independent living based upon the social model of disability.
• Disabled people must be given choice and control in all aspects of their housing.
• An equal partnership must be developed between disabled people and occupational therapists.

- There must be good liaison among agencies, with the disabled person at the centre of discussion and decision-making.
- While accessible housing is a fundamental first step, it is of little value unless wider structures in society are also made accessible.

CHAPTER 5

Conveying information through drawing

PETER ASHLEE, SYLVIA CLUTTON, SUE PENGELLY AND
JON COWDEROY

Effective communication and clarity of information are essential to ensure that adaptations are undertaken as efficiently as possible and that the completed adaptations are usable, acceptable and appropriate for individuals' needs. Drawing is an important method which can be used to promote informed discussion and convey specific information throughout the whole adaptation process, from considering options and designing the plan to undertaking the building work. If used appropriately, drawing can promote clear communication between all members of the team, including the service user and personnel from a broad range of technical and professional backgrounds. As members of this team, it is important for occupational therapists to be able to understand and communicate through drawing.

The concept of interpreting and presenting drawings of adaptations will be new to some students and early practitioners. This chapter aims to raise awareness and understanding of a range of drawing techniques which are available to beginners, demystify the experience and explore the type of information which it is important to convey to all parties. The range of drawing techniques introduced in this chapter includes templates, sketch plans and computer-aided design.

Introduction

Why are drawings needed?

An OT working in housing initially needs spatial awareness and imagination to create ideas for potential adaptations, but at some point these ideas will need to be translated into a schematic representation which can be put down on paper to be shared with the service user and other professionals. This plan is vital in the process of appraising options, considering construction issues and dealing with spatial or resource limitations and may well be altered as the decision process progresses. Drawings are useful in the problem-solving process as they prevent passing too rapidly from a suggested solution to implementing an ill-thought-out plan. A draft scale drawing of the existing dwelling can present an opportunity to make an objective analysis of the layout so that potential changes can be made and visualised on paper first, and discussed in detail before a definitive plan is formulated, evaluated and agreed.

Drawings are used between members of the team as an essential means of communication; so it is important that OTs learn the basics of the language used by architects and builders. They must be able to read, understand the technical language and critically appraise the information shown in a technical drawing, using their own professional expertise to focus on aspects of the design or adaptation which relate to how the person using it will interact successfully with it both now and in the future.

> The importance of understanding plans cannot be under-estimated. Spotting the problems and pitfalls as early as possible and suggesting solutions is of immense value to ensure a smooth transition from conception to completion. (Dodd, 1998, p. 168)

Once finalised, plans form the basis from which the agreed building work is undertaken and can be used instead of, or in conjunction with, written specifications. They, therefore, provide a crucial link between the design and construction phases of adaptation work.

Beyond the professional and team-working incentives to be able to understand and communicate through drawings, political and organisational policies also encourage this form of working. While operating within a best-value framework in which performance and service delivery are rated and evaluated in order to improve social services locally, local authority elected members and OT managers rely on OTs to thoroughly assess, plan and evaluate their completed work as efficiently and effectively as possible. The homeowner's consent, and the OT's input, must also be documented accurately, clearly and concisely, to avoid the risk of time-consuming and expensive complaints and legal challenges, which inevitably follow as a consequence of the provision of unsatisfactory adaptations. Drawings should be used to record details of the agreed adaptation and be backed up by written evidence of the OT's clinical reasoning and justification for requesting specific features in an adaptation based on the service user's assessed need. Drawing can, therefore, be used to help achieve efficient and effective working and recording, which are required by the organisation.

If a picture really can paint a thousand words, then an appropriate drawing must be a very effective form of communication. Drawings can be used by occupational therapists in housing to convey clear information which can help to:

- provide a vision of potential options;
- promote informed discussion and decision-making;
- evaluate the various options;
- gain agreement for the best proposed option;
- design a detailed plan;
- aid collaborative working;
- achieve a parity of expectations among the team members;
- record the agreed intervention accurately and concisely;
- provide accurate specific information for building work;
- save time and avoid costly mistakes;
- avoid complications arising from misunderstandings;
- attain a successful outcome for the service user.

What can go wrong if drawings are not used?

Clear communication and clarity of information are essential throughout the adaptation process to prevent misinterpretations, mistakes and the need for adaptations to be revised. Problems can result when this level of collaboration does not occur. Mistakes can occur when OTs fail to share adequate information in the form of clear drawings and specifications as this can result in unnecessary delays, disruption and expense as Case study 5.1 demonstrates.

Case study 5.1: Mr P
Mr P lived in one of four flats built around a courtyard. He mobilised with a wheelchair and needed to have a ramp built into the courtyard to enable him to access his home. The properties were owned by the local authority, whose policy stated that the housing department would arrange adaptations to communal areas.

The OT mistakenly assumed that the housing department employed surveyors who were aware of the individual needs of disabled people and had knowledge of relevant current building regulations. The brief to the housing department consisted of a written request to build a 'wheelchair ramp'.

The resultant work demonstrated that the brief had not been detailed enough. The ramp initially constructed by the housing department builder covered one-half of the existing steps, making them difficult for other ambulant tenants to use, and at a gradient of approximately 1:4 (25 per cent), the ramp was too steep for the service user to climb or descend in his wheelchair.

The situation had to be reviewed, and was only resolved when the OT submitted a detailed drawing of a ramp suitable for use by wheelchair users, with design considerations including an acceptable gradient, headroom, width, handrails, landings and guardings. The ramp was subsequently built so that the service user was able to use it safely and it no longer provided an obstacle for the other tenants.

In summary, mistakes can occur when there is a lack of clarity in communication between members of the team as a result of misinterpretation, incorrect assumptions or a lack of understanding of the skills and responsibilities of others. Confusion leads to technical faults which have to be rectified by the builder, creating delays and resulting in cost implications for the local authority. Poor information exposes the service user to the stress of having to endure repeated building work causing a lack of confidence in the OT profession and complaints to the local authority OT department. Getting it right for the service user first time is an important principle.

A range of drawing techniques can be adopted to help convey information clearly and avoid these problems. The choice of drawing techniques to illustrate the adaptations required will vary from case to case, depending on the person or persons for whom they are intended and the type and complexity of the information to be shared. These factors will be considered in the following sections before introducing the range of drawing techniques, including computer-aided designs, which are available for OTs to use.

Who are the drawings intended for?

OTs need to be able to provide suitable drawings which can be understood by service users and convey the required information to the broad range of personnel involved in the adaptation process. When considering what type of drawing is most appropriate to use with each recipient, it is useful to consider their background knowledge, their familiarity with interpreting drawn information and the type of information which they require.

The service user

Within the theory base of citizenship, the service user's need for clear information and communication is paramount. Modernising Social Services (DoH, 1998) emphasises the importance of developing systems which encourage a user-centred approach in public services, while COT (2005) requires OTs to practise with a client-centred focus.

For this to become a reality in adaptation work, the service user or advocate must be central to identifying the problem, clear about what is being proposed, able to contribute to the design stage and able to question and monitor throughout the whole process. If drawings are to be used to promote this client-centred approach, consideration should be given to the format and the method by which the material is presented to service users and their families, based on an understanding of how they will interpret and utilise the information.

The type of drawing that many service users would find most useful may not be the same as that expected by an architect, surveyor or builder. If all discussions were based on detailed technical plans, this could alienate some service users from the process rather than encourage their active participation. Three-dimensional drawings, which are less technical but easier to understand than two-dimensional plans, can be useful forms of drawing to help service users visualise how their home will be altered, but would not be technical enough to describe all building requirements.

Service users often view proposed adaptations to their home as a major, unfamiliar event and may feel restricted in participating in decision-making by their limited experience or knowledge of building work. Illustrations can be used to overcome these problems and are most effective if they are clearly explained and people are allowed time to examine them and ask questions about aspects they do not understand. Once they can visualise the proposed adaptation to their home, the service user and their family become more fully informed and empowered to participate in discussions on a more equal basis.

Service users should have access to a copy of the drawings and the written design specification, particularly if there is likely to be a time delay in the OT making recommendations and the work being undertaken. It is important that both service user and OT have copies for monitoring purposes, since by the time the work begins the recommending OT may no longer be involved. An example of partnership working and empowerment through a service user's access to information is given below.

Case study 5.2: Mrs S
Details of a proposed shower adaptation were sent to Mrs S and her husband. The housing association which owned their property started to carry out the work, but were not completing it in accordance with the OT's specification. As the couple had a copy of the proposals which they understood, they were able to ensure that the work was corrected in line with the original proposals.

Mrs S reported:

If we hadn't had the drawings, the shower wouldn't have looked the way it now does. The shower unit was being put too high for me to reach and the chair [shower seat] would have been fitted at the wrong height. We got it done right in the end thanks to your details.

Other personnel involved with adaptations

In order to complete an adaptation, OTs need to liaise with many staff across a range of departments and organisations, all of whom have varying technical expertise and knowledge of building standards and disability issues. They require different types of information for a range of diverse purposes including being involved in the design process, approving the adaptation, authorising funding and having sufficient details to undertake the required building work.

During the design process, an OT needs to be able to consult with technical experts in order to explore the feasibility of different options. To do this effectively it is useful for them to be able to sketch their requirements. Following the brief from the OT, an architect or surveyor is employed to provide technical drawings for complex adaptations. It is common practice that a joint meeting is arranged to share concerns and check understanding, and confirm that all the features which are required by the service user are incorporated into the technical drawing and design. In this way the technician and health professional collaborate to produce a meaningful plan for the service user.

Since adaptation work is undertaken by a range of specialist building and design professionals, it is expected that any drawings of an adaptation should be able to convey information effectively from one discipline to another. It should never be assumed that written adaptation proposals are understood and interpreted in the same way by members of different disciplines. Given that each discipline may view the same situation from a different perspective, drawings can provide a common language to avoid the danger of misinterpretation.

It is sometimes necessary, for funding purposes, for OT recommendations for adaptations to be authorised by staff who are administrators rather than experts in either disability or building issues. The type of drawing supplied to them needs to be clear and appropriate to avoid any unnecessary time delays in this approval process. In the case study above, a separate sketch plan of Mrs S's existing bathroom alongside a plan of the proposed adaptation were sent to the housing association, which enabled the housing officer involved to understand the requisition and to give prompt permission for the works to go ahead.

Various organisations are responsible for ensuring that adaptation work is completed according to specifications. These can include housing associations and public sector housing departments, which may not have in-house adaptation services specialising in adaptation work or staff who are familiar with the range of equipment on the market to meet the needs of disabled people. OTs also liaise with home improvement agencies (HIAs), which support older, disabled and vulnerable homeowners to remain in their own homes by helping them carry out repairs, improvements and adaptations to their properties. They often employ technical officers and contract work out to specialist surveyors/architects and local authority approved builders. They require clear detailed drawings from the OT backed up by extremely detailed design specifications which list the exact model of all the equipment recommended, a list of special features required and contact details for the suppliers of that equipment.

> **Case study 5.3: Mrs V**
> During an OT visit to Mrs V, it was recognised that it would only be feasible to adapt the rear access to her council property. This would require permission from the local housing authority to construct a path across a patch of communal grassland and modify the railings to create an opening. Consideration would need to be given to the impact of this work on the safety and convenience of other tenants. In compliance with current building regulations a ramp of over three metres in length would have been necessary to bridge the existing steps; as there were only 640 mm of length available, constructing a simple ramp was not a feasible option. Careful examination of the site resulted in the production of three-dimensional drawings which included measurements taken at the site. These drawings were used to convey the information required in the requisition to the housing department, builders and Mrs V. They enabled the team to discuss and make successful decisions away from the site as the necessary information was available.

In the interests of the service users, OTs should familiarise themselves with the information needs of the organisations and professionals they find themselves working alongside to ensure that the team works effectively during both the design and the building stages of the adaptation process.

Type and complexity of information

Another factor which will influence what methods of drawing are selected is the type of information which needs to be conveyed, especially the level of complexity of that information and the technical accuracy required. This is mainly influenced by the type of work recommended, and it is important that the method of drawing selected is consistent with the complexity of the information which needs to be conveyed. A professionally produced architect's plan would be disproportionate to the requirements of the installation of a grab rail, while an extension could not be undertaken from a simple sketch.

Minor adaptations

The most straightforward works normally undertaken are minor adaptations, the majority of which are support and hand rails, but also include the installation of long, shallow steps for people who use walking frames, non-complex ramps for attendant-propelled wheelchair users or door entry systems.

Based on their assessment of the individual, the OT will need to convey relatively simple but accurate information to ensure that the minor adaptation is installed as required for the service user. They often have direct contact with a builder who requires straightforward information, in the case of hand rails this includes the type and measurement of the rail, the exact position of where the rail is to be fitted and an idea, where possible, of the type of surface onto which it is to be mounted. Feedback from the fitter is essential, as this will highlight any technical difficulties in fitting the rail in

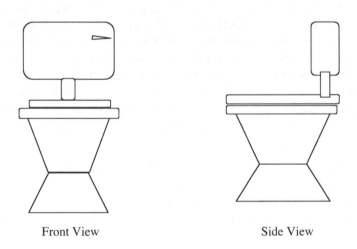

Front View   Side View

Specifications for builders:

	Right side facing	Left side facing
Number and type of rails		
Length of rails		
Height of rails from floor		
Distance of rails from wall behind toilet		
Horizontal, vertical, oblique position		

Type of fixing (i.e. to brick, wooden frame, concrete) ....

Figure 5.1.1 Templates for minor adaptations: Toilet rails.

the recommended position. Following this, the original plan may need to be amended, for example by changing the type of rail used from a wall-mounted support rail to a floor-mounted one or by repositioning it altogether.

In this situation the use of template drawings is sufficient to convey the information required. A template for minor adaptation work is a ready-made pattern/drawing of a location in the house where rails are regularly requested, for example beside steps, stairs, toilets, beds and baths.

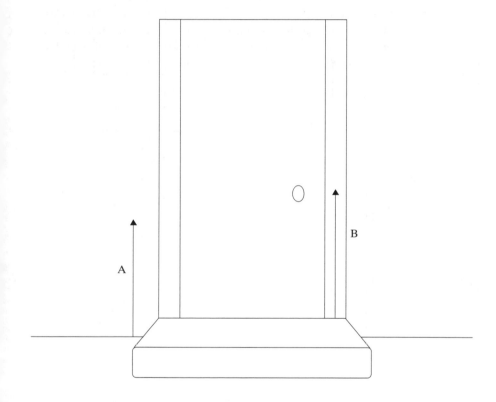

Specifications for builders:

	Right side ascending	Left side ascending
Number and type of rails		
Length of rails		
Height of rails from ground (A)		
Height of rails from step (B)		
Distance of rails away from wall		

Type of fixing (i.e. to brick, wooden frame, concrete)....................................

Figure 5.1.2 Templates for minor adaptaions: Door access.

Additional details and specific measurements need to be added to record the requirements for each individual situation. Figure 5.1 shows three examples of templates which can be drawn on a computer using basic drawing packages and are sufficient to convey the information required for the majority of minor adaptations.

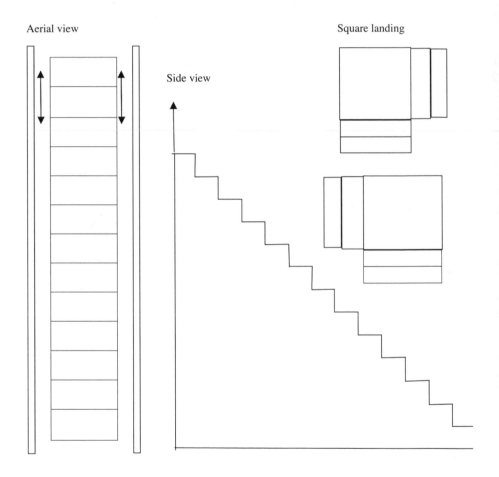

Aerial view

Square landing

Side view

Specifications for builders:

	Right side ascending	Left side ascending
Number of rails		
Length of rails		
Height of rails from floor		
Length of horizontal rails at top of stairs		
Length of horizontal rails at bottom of stairs		

Type of wall...

Figure 5.1.3 Templates for minor adaptations: Stair rails.

Case study 5.4: Mr F
Mr F had vulnerable standing balance and he had difficulty with sitting to standing, and standing while pulling up his lower garments, requiring the help of care staff. The installation of a suitably positioned support rail, and a modification to the existing toilet following clear specifications from a template, enabled him to access the toilet with dignity and deal with his dressing needs independently.

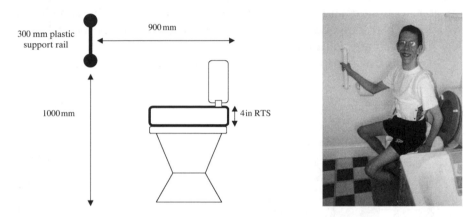

Figure 5.2 Template requisition and photograph of completed work.

Major adaptations

At the other end of the scale, when a major adaptation is identified as being necessary to meet needs, the type and complexity of the information which needs to be conveyed would make it reasonable to expect that more detailed drawings are called for. Sketch plans, scale plans, elevations and in some cases perspective drawings are more appropriate when more complex adaptation work is required. While an OT may not be required to draw to the same standard as an architect, they will need to be able to convey detailed information on the specific features required by a service user taking account of a broad range of issues identified during assessment. They will also need to be able to interpret and evaluate detailed plans.

An example of someone with complex needs, requiring detailed specifications, would be a child with severe physical and learning disabilities who displayed challenging behaviour, variable muscle tone and a vulnerable sitting balance and experienced incontinence and epilepsy. Serious thought would need to be given to detailed recommendations for major adaptations in consultation with his or her family and other significant professionals. Several specialist manufacturers would need to be involved in trials of equipment, for example hoists and bath equipment. The specific features of equipment, space requirements and safety considerations should all be incorporated into the OT's composite vision of the proposed adaptation and presented in detail to an architect. The architect would then draw a sketch plan of the proposed adaptation which would be a working document to form the focus of subsequent discussions with relevant members of the team. The OT would need to be able to interpret these drawings, evaluate them and be able to recognise when a particular configuration in an adaptation would not work for this individual service user. The OT should also be able to understand technical language to check that the schedule of works which accompanies the drawings for a major adaptation matches the features which are required by the service user in an adaptation.

An example of a proposed plan for major adaptation work is shown below.

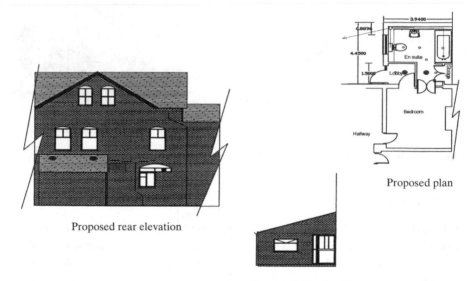

Proposed plan

Proposed rear elevation

Proposed side elevation

Figure 5.3 Proposed plan and elevation for major adaptation. Plan supplied by Ian Bown, Chartered Building Consultant.

This plan is used as the focus for further discussion, including the position of a hoist. When all parties agree, amendments are made and a definitive plan is produced.

Drawing techniques

Moving beyond the use of pre-prepared templates explored in relation to minor adaptations, there are several other techniques, using pencil and paper or a computer, which OTs can select depending on who the drawings are intended for and the complexity of the information to be conveyed. OTs are encouraged to become familiar with the whole range of drawing techniques so they can select the most appropriate one for each occasion.

Scale drawing

The concept of drawing to scale can be simply described as a means of transferring the information to be conveyed from real size to a size with which it is convenient to work, and representing that on a piece of paper of a suitable size.

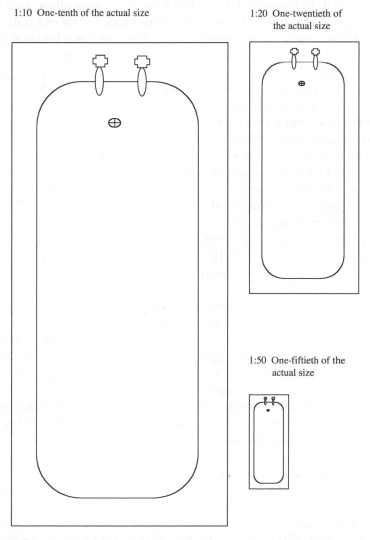

Figure 5.4 Representation of scale drawings of a bath, plan view.

The OT may be considering adapting a particular room, taking into account its fitments, fittings and space, or may be looking at the whole building and how the user will gain access to it or move around inside it, or looking at more than one building and the relationship between the buildings. The scale selected will vary depending on the size of what needs to be represented, the detail which needs to be shown and how much can be fitted on the size of the piece of paper used. If the intention is to make a drawing of a room, it is clearly not feasible to draw it as real-life size in a scale of 1:1 because the paper would need to be the size of the room, and even at a scale of 1:2 the paper would still be too big to be practical. In practice a scale of 1:20 is adopted as an appropriate scale for drawing a specific room in a property, and 1:50 for a complete property. An example of how features would appear scaled down can be demonstrated by considering a regular bath. While the actual bath measured 172 cm long and 74 cm wide, it would be too large to be drawn on the paper at a scale of 1:1. Figure 5.4 represents it drawn to scales of approximately 1:10, 1:20 and 1:50.

When annotating drawings (which involves writing specific dimensions on the plans), design professionals and builders use metric measurements as this is the accepted system in the building industry. The convention is to use metric measures on plans, using millimetres rather than centimetres (Thorpe, 1994). It is therefore advisable for OTs to draw to scale using metric measurements in compliance with the standard to improve communication and mutual understanding. The exception to this would be when communicating with older service users when consideration should be given to converting the metric measurements to the imperial measurements on the plans if they understand feet and inches better.

A retractable metal tape measure and a scale ruler are essential tools for the OT working in housing. Both are needed to enable them to draw to scale and can be purchased from any good stationers. While OTs may initially be apprehensive about using scale rulers, fears can be dispelled when it is realised that most of the scales on the ruler are hardly ever used. The 1:20 and the 1:50 scales are most commonly used. The 1:20 scale is used to pay attention to detail and particular features or fitments in a room, whereas 1:50 provides the scale of the rooms in relation to each other as well as the building's location and access. Repeated practice using the scale ruler increases confidence in its use until it is eventually taken for granted as an essential tool to convey clear information.

The simplified representation of a scale ruler in Figure 5.5 shows the most commonly used scales with measurements given in millimetres and metres.

The left-hand side indicates the scale, with the 1:1 scale measuring out at 10 mm intervals in real space. When the 0 line is placed at one end of a line in a plan drawn to 1:20 scale and its other end corresponded with the line marked 600 on the 1:20 scale of the ruler that would indicate that

1:1	0	10	20	30	40	50	60	70	80	90	100	110	120	130
1:20	0	200	400	600	800	1000	1200	1400	1600	1800	2000	2200	2400	2600
1:50	0		1m		2m		3m		4m		5m		6m	

Figure 5.5 Representation of a scale ruler to show the three most commonly used scales.

the line represented 600 mm in real space. Likewise, if the 0 is placed at one end of a line in a 1:50 plan and the other end registered 4 m on the 1:50 scale, this would indicate that the line in the plan corresponded to a length of 4 m in real space. This is important for OTs to understand as it will enable them to evaluate whether adequate space has been incorporated into the proposed plans for adaptations.

Plans and elevations

- A *plan* is a *bird's eye* view, that is the view looking directly down on an object. Plans show the length and width and can be drawn to scale and all critical dimensions can be added.
- An *elevation* is a *person's eye* view or the view looking directly across the room. While in theory elevations can be drawn from any one of the four sides of a room, in practice they are either side or end views. Elevations show length and height and can be drawn to scale and all critical dimensions can be added.

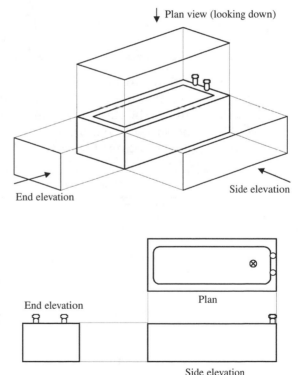

Figure 5.6 Plan and elevation of a bath.

Figure 5.6 demonstrates how a bath would be represented as a plan and as two different elevations.

Exercise example 5.1
This example demonstrates how to draw a plan and elevation of a table measuring 1800 mm long and 900 mm wide (1.8 m × 90 cm) in a scale of 1:20.

Take a scale ruler, place it horizontally on a page and draw a line between 0 and 1800 using the 1:20 scale. Draw both ends of the table at right angles to your original line by using the same scale to measuring from 0 to 900. Join up the lines to make a rectangle which represents a scale plan of the table.

This is what the *plan* should look like:

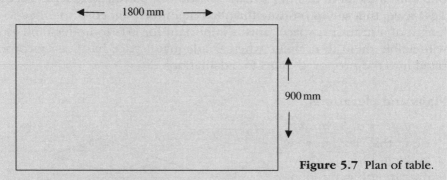

Figure 5.7 Plan of table.

Other information can be conveyed via an elevation, including the height of the table (800 mm) and the position of the legs from the edge of the table (50 mm). The thickness of the table top and the width of the legs could also be shown if required.

This is what the *elevation* should look like:

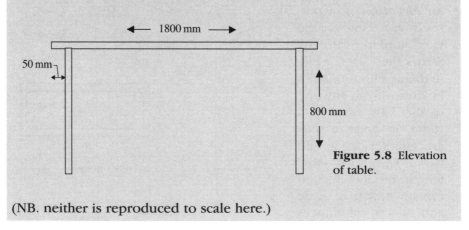

Figure 5.8 Elevation of table.

(NB. neither is reproduced to scale here.)

Repeated practice representing a range of objects to scale from these two perspectives is the best way to familiarise oneself with this drawing technique.

Plans and elevations are views from an imaginary fixed point. For example, on the drawings of the bathroom below, the viewer would be looking down from just below the top of the window. The place to position the viewer for the elevation depends on what the designer wants to show. For example, if the OT intends to take the bath out or show the position of an overbath shower, the viewer does not need to see the basin in the elevation, but does need to be able to see the full length of the bath from the side. In this instance, the section for the elevation shown in the second drawing was taken between the edge of the basin and the edge of the bath, as indicated by the arrows drawn on the plan below. This is described as 'a section through two fixed points'.

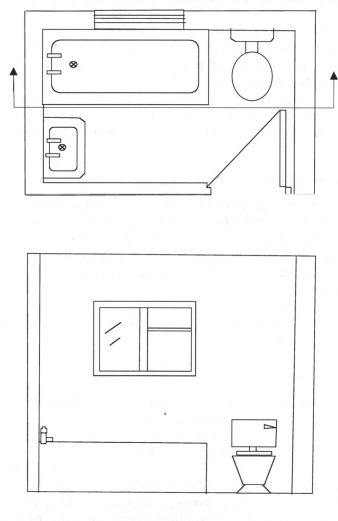

Figure 5.9 Plan and front elevation of a bathroom.

This figure also demonstrates how plans and elevations can be drawn together so that they are in line with each other. This has advantages for the person doing the drawing and the person reading the drawing. The person doing the drawing can run the lines directly up or down, or to the side if necessary, without having to measure them again. The person reading the drawing makes a direct visual correlation between the two views so that the positioning of objects is clear.

Advantages of plans and elevations

- This is the standard method of conveying information within the building industry and is a convention and a 'language' shared by all involved.
- Crucial information can be conveyed clearly and accurately so that there is no question of ambiguity.
- All necessary annotation and dimensions can be added to the drawing, with an attached written specification.
- When there are problems with access to a property, or in circumstances where it is not clear from an initial assessment what course of action should be taken, a scale plan can be extremely useful in illustrating and appraising options.

Disadvantages of plans and elevations

- The conventions and shared language used by professionals in plans can exclude service users from meaningful discussion and input to the proposals; so they should not be used in isolation.
- As plans are often amended over time, confusion can arise when agents work from different drafts. To avoid this, serial drafts of plans should be dated and signed.
- Formal drawings and plans can be unnecessarily time-consuming for small alterations or minor adaptations when alternatives such as templates can be used.

Isometric drawings

Isometric drawing is a means of combining the *plan and two elevations* on one drawing. It is not possible to draw in this style entirely to scale because the lines coming towards the observer are foreshortened, giving the impression that the drawing is in perspective. Isometric drawings are not quite as technically informative as perspective drawings. However, as a picture of the proposal, they are easy to draw, they give the service user a clear, visual sense of the finished work and dimensions can be accurately marked. It is also possible to obtain the correct proportion by drawing the end elevation to scale.

The rule for constructing isometric drawings is that all of the lines are either vertical or at an angle of roughly 30 degrees.

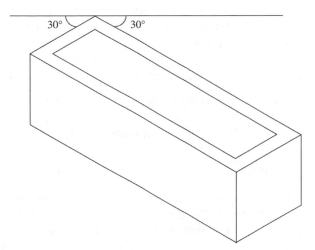

30°   30°

Figure 5.10 Isometric drawing of a bath.

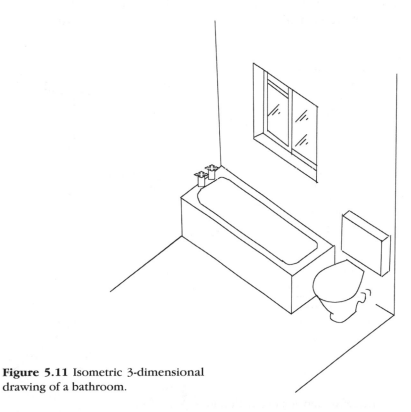

Figure 5.11 Isometric 3-dimensional drawing of a bathroom.

Advantages of isometric drawings

- Instantly clear what is proposed to experts and non-experts.
- Most necessary dimensions and annotations can be added easily.
- They are quick and easy to draw, and can be done during the assessment at the service user's home.

Disadvantages of isometric drawings

- As only two elevations can be seen, it may not be possible to draw all of the details required.
- It is not possible to draw entirely to scale.

Perspective drawings

Perspective drawing is a means of combining the *plan and three elevations* on one drawing. The designer cannot draw this entirely to scale because the lines coming towards them are foreshortened to create the illusion of depth. However, as a picture of what is proposed, it is clear and dimensions can be accurately marked. It is possible to obtain the correct proportion by drawing the end elevation to scale. Perspective drawings are easy to draw and are visually as well as technically very informative.

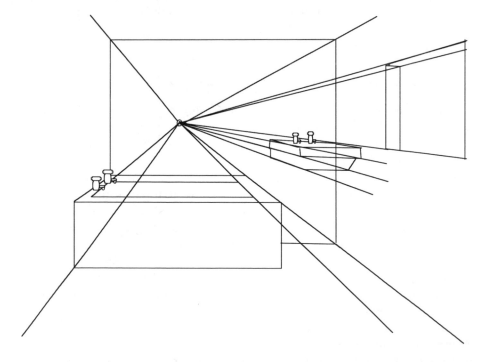

Figure 5.12 Perspective drawing of a bathroom.

The rule for constructing perspective drawings is that all of the lines going away from the designer lead to one imaginary vanishing point, which can be placed wherever required. If the person for whom the proposed adaptations are being planned is a tall ambulant person, the vanishing point can be positioned relatively high. Alternatively, it can be positioned lower to provide the perspective for a wheelchair user. When the vanishing point is determined, all lines from the objects in the drawing will lead to it and away from it. For example, in the figure below, the designer drew the lines from the vanishing point to the edge of the bath, and then brought them towards themself to show the sides of the bath. The length of the sides of the bath on the drawing were chosen for appearance, not accuracy, as it is not possible to draw this to scale. All the other objects on the drawing such as basin, walls and windows also lead to the vanishing point.

Advantages of perspective drawings

* Instantly clear what is proposed to experts and non-experts.
* All necessary dimensions and annotations can be added.

Disadvantages of perspective drawings

* More time-consuming than some other types of drawing and not necessarily practical when designing minor adaptations.
* Not possible to draw entirely to scale.

Computer-aided design

Computer-aided design (CAD) is an increasingly popular and ever more accessible medium for achieving clear, accurate designs to support OT recommendations for adaptations for people with disabilities. It is a fact of modern life that people have increased access to personal computers at home and in the workplace, and, when this is combined with developments in CAD software packages, it means that computer-generated diagrams are achievable and available for both service provider and service user alike. A well-constructed CAD diagram is easy to interpret, accurate to scale and can be altered and enhanced with ease. It can be rapidly accessed via email and has a professional appearance, making it an ideal tool for all parties involved in disability design and adaptation.

CAD diagrams can be constructed in two dimensions (2D), in plan or elevation format, or have more sophisticated 'walkthrough' features that give the option of viewing any aspect of a room in three dimensions (3D). Therefore, in the case of a kitchen adaptation, for example, it is possible to view the facilities from the perspective of a wheelchair user as well as from ambulant height. From the designer's perspective, CAD also allows them to cut and paste objects within a diagram at will. This means facilities including showers, baths and cookers can be picked up and 'dragged and dropped' across the diagram with ease. In short, a complex adaptation can be constructed on the computer and then reviewed from the angle of choice. Any alterations that are required can be made with the click of a mouse until the desired format is achieved. The following CAD designs include a plan of the author's existing bathroom and two 3D representations of a proposed new layout for that bathroom from two differing perspectives.

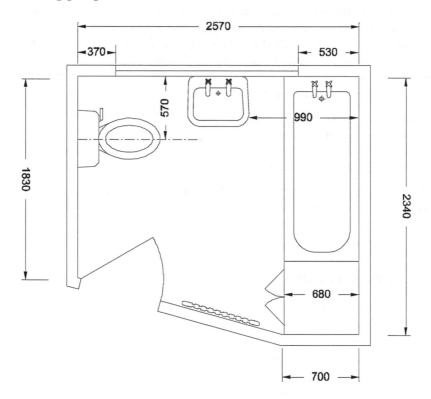

Figure 5.13 CAD plan of existing bathroom.

Another advantageous feature of CAD is the ability to reuse or recycle previous diagrams. For example, in the case of a level access shower, guidance is often sought as to where the services in the wet area should be located such as support rails, shower riser rail and seat height. A pre-constructed format can be downloaded and utilised repeatedly to show the desired layout (see figure 5.16).

All adjustments can be made for specific situations by changing the position of the services by 'dragging and dropping', as well as rotating and

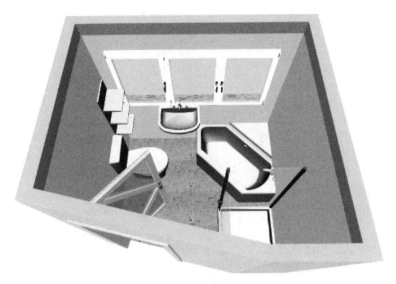

Figure 5.14 CAD 3D perspective of proposed bathroom seen from above.

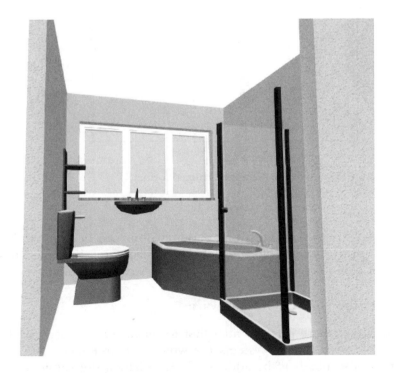

Figure 5.15 CAD 3D perspective of proposed bathroom viewed from wheelchair height.

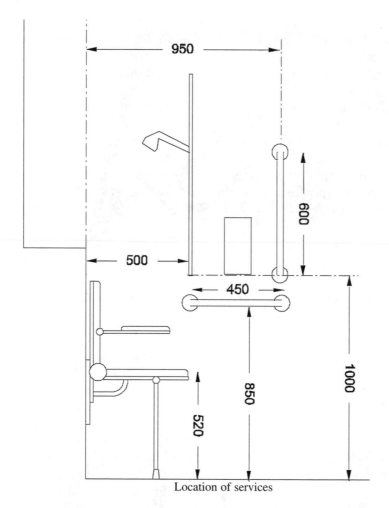

Location of services

Figure 5.16 CAD downloaded pre-constructed format.

mirroring as required and the new dimensions can be applied. This, of course, improves time efficiency as new diagrams do not need to be drawn or constructed from scratch with every recommendation.

Selecting the correct CAD software

As with all software it is essential first to make sure that any package is compatible with the PC systems for which it is intended. The issue of copyright also needs to be addressed, especially if the software is to be used in an office or departmental setting. The cost and complexity of the packages available today vary widely. Some of the early basic systems can be purchased for a few pounds, while the more sophisticated packages designed for architectural purposes can run as high as four figures. By rule of thumb the more complex any given CAD software is, the more it costs. It is advisable to determine what complexity of diagram is required and purchase appropriately to that requirement.

It is also important to examine the 'symbol library' of a desired package. This is a collection of pre-constructed objects (such as shower trays and support rails), as well as surfaces and templates that can be dropped into a diagram. It is possible for an OT to create their own symbols, especially for 2D format, by constructing and saving them in the library; however, for ease of operation it is best to have the desired symbols already available.

CAD training

Like word processing software, CAD programs tend to share common features of operation. However, even the most basic program can prove daunting at first sight, and the various functions are not obvious to the untrained eye. It is, therefore, advisable to spend time learning the necessary skills to operate these systems. They all come with their own 'help' folders and most have in-built tutorials or training programs. It is strongly recommended that these are followed carefully as this will prevent future frustration and improve speed of operation once the features are properly understood. CAD training can also be undertaken at colleges and evening classes, and peripatetic instructors are available.

The first attempts at constructing detailed plans will be a slow process as newly acquired skills are applied. It is important to persevere at this stage and not be discouraged. The more practice the OT has, the quicker they will become, so that before long they will be constructing professional detailed diagrams at a fraction of the speed of the hand-drawn image. Once they are familiar with their use OTs will find that using CAD is a fast and efficient method of providing clear, accurate and detailed drawings for adaptations, which can be understood by professionals and non-professionals alike.

Conclusion

When drawing techniques are selected and used appropriately, they can promote effective communication – which is essential throughout the whole adaptation process. The ability to understand plans and communicate through a range of drawing techniques will enable an OT to communicate effectively with both service users and other personnel involved in adaptation work drawn from a broad range of technical and professional backgrounds. Drawing and the use of CAD are important skills for OTs to acquire and have profound implications for achieving successful outcomes for service users.

This chapter has aimed to help the reader to become aware of the importance of drawing to convey information within housing and to provide an initial introduction to a range of techniques available to do this. It also sought to provide them with the motivation to explore this area further as it is recognised that simply reading about practical skills is not sufficient to obtain those skills. A potter does not acquire their skills through reading but by learning from experience. The reader is therefore encouraged to practise the techniques discussed in the chapter and to investigate training opportunities which would help them to acquire these drawing skills and gain confidence in using them to convey information. The process of researching, experimenting with, reflecting on and evaluating new techniques to improve communication through drawings should be an ongoing process among OTs working in housing.

Key points

- Drawing is an important communication tool which can be used to convey clear and accurate information which is necessary throughout the whole adaptation process.
- Once they are familiar with producing and interpreting drawings, OTs can use these skills to share their understanding of housing problems, provide images of possible solutions and evaluate proposed adaptations.
- The type of drawings used must be understood by the service user, and appropriate for the needs of other members of the team.
- Three-dimensional drawings are usually easier for service users and other non-technically trained people to understand, while two-dimensional plans are indispensable to convey detailed technical information.
- The ability to draw to scale and familiarise themselves with CAD is a key area for CPD for all OTs working in housing.

Acknowledgements

Thanks to Becky Ennion, Peter Broadhead, Chris and Peter Weston, science and IT specialists, for advice on drawing. Thanks to Ian Bown, Chartered Building Consultant, for building plan.

CHAPTER 6

Access standards: evolution of inclusive housing

PARAIG O'BRIEN

Occupational therapists in collaboration with disabled people and design professionals have a valued role to play in the evaluation and development of inclusive design standards. This chapter offers the reader an opportunity to reflect on the models and approaches from occupational therapy practice which interface with environmental design. The chapter also examines the principles and application of selected design approaches to occupational therapy practice. Having explored the development of conceptual thinking in this area, the focus moves to a critical appraisal of actual benchmark design guidance relating to housing. The standards applying to both 'general needs' and wheelchair standard housing are mapped out to allow a comparison of design elements and consider their application to the needs of disabled people. The chapter highlights the accelerating movement towards inclusive design in housing and promotes a debate as to what constitutes best practice.

Introduction

In historical terms, it comes as a considerable surprise to many people to discover that, despite the presence of large numbers of disabled people in or, indeed, marginalised within our society (Oliver, 1990), there is relatively little archaeological or literary evidence of their needs being systematically considered in the design of buildings or housing until very recently.

For example, the design of the modern-day bath has actually evolved little since the Minoan Dynasty in Crete (which collapsed around 1450 BC). The tradition of the bath was adopted by the Greeks of the Mycenaean period and later the Romans. Bathing became less popular in the Middle Ages and only really re-emerged in the nineteenth century, 'when it remained as the fundamental device for body cleansing' (Mullick, 2001, ch. 42, p. 3). Today occupational therapists spend much of their professional expertise helping elderly and disabled people to overcome the inherent constraints of maintaining personal hygiene in the bathtub, which, in design terms, is an inherently flawed product.

The expectations of what a home should provide have broadened over time. In earlier times one of the main priorities was to create a defensible home. The Norman castle, for example, was often located on a steep hill or manmade mound, had narrow windows, doors located above ground level and spiral staircases to make it more defensible; such features were specifically included to make buildings inaccessible. The need for security has been maintained with additional requirements for accessibility and usability.

The world's first National Disability Access standard A1117.1 was established in the USA in 1961 (ASA, 1961). Specific standards for housing and public buildings in the UK emerged with Selwyn Goldsmith's 1963 publication *Designing for the Disabled*. The history of access guidance for the design of dwellings is therefore a short one, but nevertheless it is an area where considerable advances have occurred in recent years. These advances have been both ideological and technological.

This chapter explores conceptual changes and developments in design standards which have been significant in this drive towards inclusive housing.

The drivers for change

A number of catalysts are motivating society to give greater priority to the creation of inclusive housing in recent years.

- *Demographics*: the UK population is ageing; by 2003 16 per cent of the UK population was over 65 representing a 3 per cent increase since 1971 (National Statistics, 2005), and there is a direct correlation between age and disability (McCoy and Smith, 1992).
- *Legislation*: the disability movement has been influential in spearheading movement from welfare to rights-based legislation (Oliver, 1990). The rights to assessment (including housing needs) for disabled people and carers have been strengthened in recent years.
- *Social policy*: there is increasing recognition of the important role accessible housing plays in terms of social inclusion/integration (Greater London Authority, 2004).
- *Improved needs assessment*: the growing number of community-based occupational therapists are systematically identifying unmet housing need in this area.

- *Accident prevention*: the design features of housing are often associated with home accidents (DTI, 2001); therefore improved housing design can play a substantial role in home accident prevention (Blythe et al., 2002).
- *Economics*: expenditure on home adaptations continues to rise sharply in many countries (Department of Health, Social Services and Public Safety/Northern Ireland Housing Executive, 2002). Disabled Facilities Grant (DFG) expenditure in England alone rose from £56m in 1997/1998 to £101.5m in 2004/2005 (ODPM, 2004b), leading to an increased awareness of the importance of considering accessibility in new-build housing.

As society has developed new concepts of equality of opportunity, these have in turn influenced legislation, design approaches and the access standards of our housing and public-built environment.

How can occupational therapists influence change?

There are some central questions for occupational therapists to consider in relation to housing design.

- What occupational therapy approaches underpin our core values and beliefs in the field of housing for people with disabilities?
- How are these approaches reflected in terms of housing design?
- How inclusive or universal are our design standards for the full range of potential users, i.e. children, ambulant disabled people, independent wheelchair users, assisted wheelchair users, people with sensory loss, cognitive impairments and people from minority ethnic backgrounds?
- How can occupational therapists engage with service users and design professionals to ensure that these design standards genuinely meet the real and diverse needs of society?

Occupational therapists have much to offer in the evaluation and development of design standards in housing for disabled people. Increasingly, collaborative research and development involving disabled people, design professionals and occupational therapists is helping to establish good practice in this field (National Wheelchair Housing Association Group, 1997; Atkinson and Dodd, 2002; Awang, 2004; Greater London Authority, 2004; NIHE, 2004).

Table 6.1 gives a brief overview of the chronological sequence of events on both sides of the Atlantic, which are shaping design standards. There is no singular blueprint for the design of the 'ideal' home, and, despite significant advances in the last forty years, this field is set to change further, driven by changes in society, human expectations, legislation, technology and community care.

Table 6.1 The major milestones in the evolution of inclusive housing

Year	Event
1961	America develops the world's first national disability access standard A1117.1 (Public Buildings)
1967	Britain develops its first access standard CP96 (Public Buildings)
1970	Chronically Sick and Disabled Persons Act
1974	HDDOP 2/74 Mobility Housing
1975	HDDOP 2/75 Wheelchair Housing
1978	BS 5619 Design of housing for the convenience of disabled people
1988	Fair Housing Amendments Act enacted in the USA (7 access design standards)
1990	NHS & Community Care Act
1990	Americans with Disabilities Act
1992	Manual Handling Operations Regulations
1995	Disability Discrimination Act
1995	The Carers (Recognition and Services) Act
1997	Lifetime homes standards published by Joseph Rowntree Foundation (JRF)
1998	Lifetime homes standards implemented for social housing in Northern Ireland
1999	Part M Building Regulations extend to domestic dwellings for the first time
1999	Meeting Part M and Designing Lifetime Homes published by JRF
2001	BS: 8300 Design of buildings and their approaches to meet the needs of disabled people – Code of practice
2004	Adapting Homes and Housing Sight published by Welsh Assembly for people with sight loss
2005	Habinteg Wheelchair Housing Design Guide published

(Variances occur in legislation and design standards for Scotland and Northern Ireland.)

Concepts influencing housing design standards

The ideological approaches to accessible housing design have evolved rapidly in the last forty years. It is possible to track a series of health and social care concepts, which have become influential in how we both deliver care and respond to the built environment. A brief summary of these concepts will be outlined before we examine parallel concepts in the design world. The relationships between models of human need, design approaches and housing standards are outlined in Figure 6.1.

Models of human need

These concepts are presented in broadly chronological order.

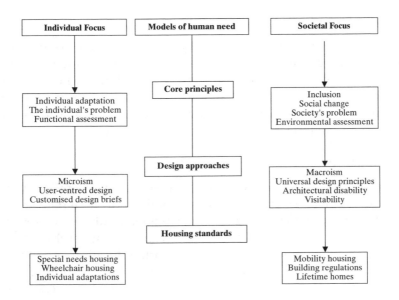

Figure 6.1 Concepts influencing housing design.

The biomedical model

This model views the individual as having a problem as a result of their medical condition, and the onus is primarily on the individual to adapt to the environment. The biomedical model has been criticised from a number of perspectives (Jones et al., 2000) as it understands disease as a categorical departure from 'normality' and often fails to offer comprehensive solutions to people with long-term and life-limiting illness. Increasingly, community occupational therapy services are moving towards the social model of disability but retain elements of the medical model where it has a role in the verification and determination of longer-term health needs, risk assessment and gate-keeping resources.

The rehabilitation model

The rehabilitation model aims to regain the previous level of function, not necessarily maximum function (Hagedorn, 1995). The biomechanical, neuro-developmental and cognitive frames of reference may be drawn on depending on the nature of the impairment. In this model one provides balanced environmental support and challenge, and the focus is on mastery of the environment. Once rehabilitation has been optimised, therapists may consider the adaptation model.

The adaptation model

This model is often significant for occupational therapists working in housing. The model involves not just environmental adaptation but personal and occupational adaptation. It is considered when maximum rehabilitation has been achieved. Adaptive approaches are focused on the environment (mechanical, architectural and aesthetic) as well as on the individual and the tasks performed.

The social model of disability

This model was developed by disability activists who identified that the core of the 'problem' rested with society not the individual (Oliver, 1990). The model proposes that social and environmental discrimination needs to be addressed so that disabled people can avail themselves of mainstream life opportunities such as transport, education, employment, access and income. The model can readily be applied to housing services where the focus is on the removal of environmental barriers to social inclusion. It is influential in the community and voluntary sector and increasingly is valued in the statutory sector, where, for example, it has been recommended as a model for housing adaptations services (ODPM/DoH, 2004).

Normalisation

This concept also offers an inclusive view of disability, and the principles have had greatest impact in the field of learning difficulties. The aim was to 'develop services to allow people to enjoy patterns of life and conditions of everyday living which are as close as possible to the regular circumstances and ways of life of society' (Nirje, 1980, p. 33). The principles are clearly outlined in John O'Brien's (1987) five main service accomplishments, which underpin many of our community services today.

- Community presence
- Choice
- Competence
- Respect
- Community participation

The adoption of these principles alongside community care principles has resulted in more people living in their own homes rather than institutions. They support choice in where to live, facilitate people to live in mainstream housing rather than in institutions and promote the importance of being part of a growing network of friends.

In parallel with these health and social care concepts comparable design concepts have emerged. It is useful to understand these concepts to aid communications with colleagues in the design professions and to create new constructs for problem-solving.

The development of design approaches

Accessibility

The term 'access' requires some exploration, as there are variant meanings in conventional dictionaries. The definitions can extend from the 'act of approaching or entering' to the 'right or privilege to approach, enter, or make use of something' (McCleoud and Hanks, 1987, p. 6).

The second definition includes the concept of being able to use facilities. In practice this is a much higher design standard than just being able to get into a building or dwelling. It is possible for a facility to be described as accessible even though it is not usable! As differential space standards are reflected in various building regulations and access guides, one must check carefully to see what level of actual usability is being described. It is interesting to note that the definition which accompanies the American National Standard (CABO/ANSI A117.1-1992) defines accessibility as a site, building or portion thereof that complies with this standard and that can be approached, entered and used by people with physical disabilities.

By contrast, the definition which accompanies Part M of the Building Regulations (1999) in the UK states that accessibility with respect to buildings or parts of buildings, means that disabled people are able to gain access. This is further defined as approach or entry only. To confuse matters later in the text, the Building Regulations also use the term 'suitable', meaning the facilities should be designed for use by disabled people.

In practice these building regulations are minimum standards only and can fall short of creating suitable facilities for all disabled users to use, for example assisted wheelchair users, people who use scooters, carers (Goldsmith, 2001) and people with sensory loss. Goldsmith (1963) also differentiates between wheelchair access and wheelchair use, with wheelchair use requiring more generous space standards.

User-centred design

The principles of user-centred design were developed by Stephen Pheasant, an ergonomist at the Royal Free Hospital in London. His work continues to be of particular relevance to occupational therapists.

The eight principles of user-centred design described by Pheasant are:

1. *It is empirical* – It seeks to base the decisions of the design process upon hard data concerning the physical and mental characteristics of human beings, their observed behaviour and their reported experiences. It is distrustful both of grand theories and intuitive judgements – except in so much as these may be used as the starting points for empirical studies.
2. *It is iterative* – It is a cyclical process in which the research phase of empirical studies is followed by a design phase, in which solutions are generated which can in turn be evaluated empirically.
3. *It is participative* – It seeks to enrol the end user of the product as an active participant in the design process.
4. *It is non-procrustean* – It deals with people, as they are not how they might be: it aims to fit the product to the user rather than vice versa.
5. *It takes account of human diversity* – It aims to achieve the best possible match for the greatest number of people.
6. *It takes due account of the user's task* – It recognises that the match between the product and the task is commonly task-specific.
7. *It is systems orientated* – It recognises the interaction between product and user takes place in the context of a bigger socio-technical system, which in turn operates within the context of economic and political systems and environmental ecosystems.
8. *It is pragmatic* – It recognises that there may be limits to what is reasonably practical in any particular case and seeks to reach the best possible outcome within the constraints imposed by these limits. (Pheasant, 1996, p. 13)

When occupational therapists draw on the ergonomic approach within the adaptation model, user-centred design offers a practical and evidence-based approach to apply ergonomic techniques systematically to design scenarios. Pheasant's anthropometric data on the UK population, stratified by age and gender, also offer practitioners in the UK a more appropriate and reliable data source than earlier data, which were largely based on American military personnel (Dreyfuss, 1959) for product and environmental design. Many occupational therapists are already using these techniques, if unconsciously. Techniques such as activity analysis and user trials are central to user-centred design and are also core techniques in occupational therapy practice. This specialised knowledge of 'the ergonomics of disability' gives occupational therapists an important role in the overall design of products and environments (see Chapter 8).

Universal design

The original principles of universal design were developed throughout the 1990s at the Centre for Universal Design at North Carolina State University. In 1995 ten principles were established which through consultation were simplified to six:

1. *Make it easy to understand* – the design should be easy to understand, regardless of the user's knowledge or language skills.
2. *Make it easy to operate* – the design should require minimum user effort and cause minimum fatigue.
3. *Communicate with the user* – the design should communicate effectively, regardless of the user's sensory abilities.
4. *Design for user error* – the design should minimise the risk of damage or injury caused by user mistakes.
5. *Accommodate a range of methods of use* – the design should allow methods of use according to the user's preferences or abilities.
6. *Allow space for access* – the design should provide ample space for approach and manoeuvring regardless of the user's body size and position. Each of these principles is also accompanied by further guidelines. (Storey, 2001, Ch. 10, p. 5)

Equitable use was added to the final version, which meant that the design should not disadvantage or stigmatise any group of users.

Universal design suggest that the built environment should reflect the needs and requirements of all building users, as well as addressing the problems experienced by people who have reduced physical, sensory and cognitive ability. The philosophy also promotes user involvement in the design process itself, and as such the term 'inclusive design' is often used to describe this more holistic approach (Luck et al., 2001).

There is a significant difference between accessibility and universal design.

> Accessibility is a function of compliance with regulations or criteria that establish a minimum level of design necessary to accommodate people with disabilities. Universal design, however, is the art and practice of design to accommodate the widest variety and number of people throughout their life-spans. (Salmen, 2001, Ch. 12, p. 1)

Universal design principles are extremely useful for occupational therapists as they incorporate both sound ergonomic and anti-discriminatory principles. Universal design also promotes holistic and inclusive thinking about the totality of human need in society.

The principles can form a framework for a design brief whether this is for an assistive technology device or design in the built environment. By considering everyone's needs early in the design brief, costly and time-consuming mistakes may be avoided later on.

The principles can also be used to evaluate the effectiveness of assistive technologies, housing or public building projects.

COTSSIH in its Research and Development Strategic Vision and Action Plan 2004 (objective 2) supports the development of research aimed at the understanding and implementation of universal design. COTSSIH members have made significant contributions to research and policy development related to the implementation and evaluation of Lifetime Homes in the UK (Blythe et al., 2002; Greater London Authority, 2004).

Applying both user-centred and universal design approaches

Occupational therapists in practice often use user-centred design approaches when formulating a brief for housing adaptations, based on the needs of a disabled person. Enhanced knowledge is required to advise on the design of public buildings, new-build schemes or an adaptation for a family where there are multiple users with varying needs; here the application of universal design approaches are valuable.

The approaches in practice can be complementary, for example by systematically building up ergonomic data using empirical research on representative populations of building users, using user-centred design approaches, it is possible to move towards the ultimate goal of achieving truly universal design for the total population.

A simple experiment demonstrates the interface between user-centred and universal design in practice. If one wanted to identify the optimal location for electrical sockets, one could identify the comfortable reach constraints of each user in a population in both a seated and standing position. By mapping out the individual optimal locations for each user (user-centred design) one can eventually identify the optimal location for the general population (universal design).

Interestingly, when one undertakes this experiment and compares the results against the current location for sockets in current Building Regulations applied to Dwellings (minimum height 450 mm above floor level, which most builders default to in practice), it is clearly not the optimal location for all users as it favours seated users over standing users, who have to stoop quite low to reach the socket. A location between 600 mm and 750 mm would be more suitable. The author would suggest that building regulations should try to reflect a universal design philosophy.

In practice one can encounter conflicting design parameters, which can be difficult to resolve to everyone's satisfaction and within finite resources. This may be evident when trying to reconcile the needs of children and adults in the same environment or when promoting cultural diversity. There may be occasions where the pragmatism of the user-centred design approach has a role when working through complex design details.

Microism and macroism

Selwyn Goldsmith (1997) coined these terms:

1. *Macroism* – 'the architect who is a macroist is someone who – when designing a building observes the treat as normal principle – does not incorporate special provision for disabled people where suitable provision will serve. His main aim is to extend the parameters of normal provision as far as they will go' (Goldsmith, 1997, p. 155).

   Goldsmith states that mobility housing was a macroist concept in that it was based on the principle of designing general needs housing in such a way as to accommodate the needs of ambulant disabled people. Macroism has strong similarities to universal design principles and was conceived in a similar timescale.

2. *Microism* by contrast assumes a 'Treat as different starting position . . . that disabled people are different . . . and that special – and sometimes exclusive – facilities should be provided for them' (ibid., p. 19)

   Goldsmith cites the unisex (and normally locked) wheelchair standard public toilet in Britain as an example of microism in practice. By contrast, disabled persons WCs are often integrated into mainstream toilet provision for the general public in countries such as the USA or in other European countries.

Opinion still differs on the application of these approaches. While many independent wheelchair users may prefer integrated WC provision, some assisted wheelchair users who have a companion of the other sex may prefer separate facilities. In practice it may be worth considering a mix of provision where possible.

Architectural disability

This concept was described by Selwyn Goldsmith as 'a version of the social model of disability' (ibid., p. 149). The concept goes a little further in that it is not confined to people with 'medical' disabilities only:

> An architecturally disabled person is a person who, when using or seeking to use a building, is confronted by an impediment which would not have been there, or would not have been so irksome, had the architect who designed the building done so in a way that was responsive to his or her particular needs. (ibid., p. 152)

Again, this concept has parallels in universal and user-centred design.

Visitability

Central to the social model of disability is the concept of social inclusion. In the context of housing one of the practical expressions of this ideal has been that housing design should not only consider the needs of the permanent occupants of the house but also friends and family who might visit. These standards also help disabled people visit their neighbours. This has led housing designers to consider a series of design features, which promote visitability.

A dwelling 'is visitable if any visitor can reach the entrance and all the facilities that a visitor is normally allowed to use' (Dodd, 1998, p. 169).

This concept has found practical expression in lifetime homes standards, which have been implemented for new-build social housing in Northern Ireland (Blythe et al., 2002), Wales (Rees and Lewis, 2003) and for all sectors in London (Greater London Authority, 2004).

Since the Building Regulations Part M was first applied to housing in 1999, basic visitability has also been promoted in all new-build housing in England and Wales. Other parts of the UK have also implemented similar building regulations. It should be remembered that visitability standards are a lesser standard than the standards that a wheelchair user would require if living in the home on a daily basis.

The Government recently launched its Decent Homes initiative (ODPM, 2004a), which plans to ensure that by 2010 all local authority and Registered Social Landlord-owned property is wind and weather tight, warm and with modern facilities. COTSSIH has argued that this is an excellent opportunity to promote visitability as existing housing stock is refurbished. There is concern that access features have not been given sufficient consideration in these plans. For example, the provision of UPVC doors may create unsuitable thresholds for many people.

Overall, as we reflect on evolving concepts in design, the general trend is towards thinking not only of the individual and their specific needs but also increasingly the carers' or families' needs within the context of the society in which they live.

There is also a movement away from considering the needs of disabled people as special or additional, which can lead to segregation and stigma. Instead, the objective is to promote social inclusion through holistic, mainstream design approaches, which consider the widest possible range of needs and design solutions, and which take a long-term view of both the human lifecycle and use of the built environment.

Having outlined the main health, social and design concepts which have influenced the movement towards accessible housing, the development of specific design standards will now be examined.

The emergence of house types and design standards

A working knowledge of the design features of various house types and design standards is essential for occupational therapists and housing providers, so that they can accurately match suitable housing to the assessed needs of disabled people. Identification of best practice in design standards and design elements is also critical when specifying housing adaptations. While this chapter will focus on standards in new-build housing, the reader is referred to *Building in Evidence: Reviewing Housing and Occupational Therapy* (Awang, 2004) for a critique of some recently published housing adaptation design guides.

The material in this chapter should be read alongside the earlier COTSSIH publication *Housing Options for Disabled People* (Bull, 1998a), in particular the chapter on 'Regulations, standards, design guides and plans' by Trevor Dodd, which gives an excellent overview of the main house types and design standards. This section therefore places greater emphasis on major developments since 1998 but outlines earlier standards so that the reader can track the evolution of the housing design process.

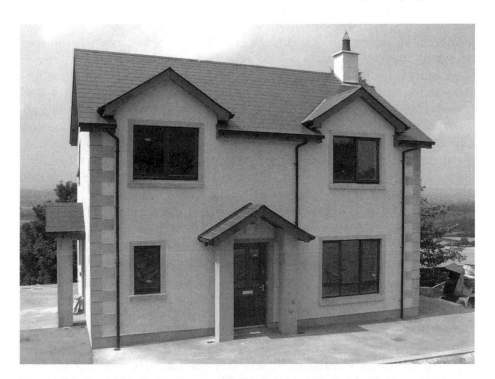

Figure 6.2 Example of a lifetime home. Photograph supplied by Habinteg, Ulster.

Because design standards applying to housing vary, there is often confusion as to what constitutes best practice. To assist the reader, charts of some of the more influential design standards have been compiled to allow a direct comparison of design elements and consider their respective suitability for disabled people. An analysis of general needs housing is followed by an exploration of variants of wheelchair standard housing. In each instance the standards are critically appraised in relation to their suitability for disabled people.

Mainstream accessible housing

This section will explore the evolution of mainstream housing by considering the developments through Mobility Housing, Lifetime Homes and the extension of Building Regulations Part M to domestic dwellings. Table 6.2 gives the reader an overview of these and makes an initial comparison between the three.

HDDOP 2/74 Mobility Housing 1974

The architect Selwyn Goldsmith developed templates for both mobility housing and wheelchair standard housing in response to the Chronically Sick and Disabled Persons Act 1970. These standards have been very influential in the design of public (social) housing since the 1970s in particular (DoE, 1974).

Mobility housing is ordinary housing built to prevailing public authority housing cost limits and space standards but designed so that it is convenient for disabled people to live in (see Table 6.2). Wheelchair access is possible to the entrance and principal rooms, and the bathroom and WC are reachable without using steps. Mobility housing is potentially suitable for all ambulant disabled people to live in, including those who use wheelchairs but are not chair-bound. The house type is also suitable for general needs housing.

Lifetime Homes 1994

The advent of lifetime homes has done much to develop the principle of designing inclusive mainstream general needs housing. The lifetime homes standards have resulted from several years of collaborative work involving the Joseph Rowntree Foundation (JRF), Habinteg Housing Association, other Housing Associations and the Access Committee for England. The very first homes were built in York in 1994. The term describes a home, which incorporates sixteen design features, which are together known as lifetime homes standards. A seventeenth standard relating to fully automatic heating systems and controls has been added in Northern Ireland. These design features can be applied to the vast majority of

Table 6.2 The evolution of mainstream accessible housing, 1974–98

Housing design element	1974 HDDOP 2/74 Mobility Housing	1997 Lifetime Homes Standards	1999 The building Regulations Approved Document M: Access and Facilities for Disabled People
Access to dwelling			
Car parking	Hard standing desirable Covered access to dwelling	Can be widened to 3,300 mm	No mandatory requirement. Driveway may form a means of approach
Paths	Not less than 1000 mm	Not less than 900 mm	900 mm width minimum
Ramp gradient	1:12 Maximum	1:12 Maximum up to 5000 mm length 1:15 if not longer than 10,000 mm 1:20 level approach	1:12 up to 5,000 mm length. 1:15 up to 10,000 mm length. 1:20 level approach
Main entrance approach	Level or ramped	Level or gently sloping	Level access 1:20 width 900 mm minimum. 1:15 < 1:20 Ramp If steeper than 1:15 see steps.
Threshold	Flush or 25 mm max upstand	Level threshold or 15 mm upstand maximum	An 'accessible' threshold – 15 mm upstand maximum
Lifts (where applicable)	1400 x 1100 mm internal dimension 750 mm clear door opening width	1400 mm (length) × 1100 mm (width)	Length 1,250 mm Width 900 mm 800 mm clear door opening width
External doors	900 mm doorset	800 mm clear opening width	775 mm clear opening width minimum
Internal circulation			
Internal doors: doorset Clear opening width	900 mm doorset	750 mm with 1200 mm corridor 800 mm with 900 mm corridor	750–800 mm clear opening width depending on direction of approach

Table 6.2 continued

Housing design element	1974 HDDOP 2/74 Mobility Housing	1997 Lifetime Homes Standards	1999 The building Regulations Approved Document M: Access and Facilities for Disabled People
Internal circulation (cont'd)			
Door hanging	Should facilitate wheelchair manoeuvre	See design guide	Outward swinging door at WC
Corridors	900 mm	900 mm minimum 1200 mm where there is a 90° turn into a 750 mm door (750 mm for short obstructions)	900 mm minimum up to 1200 mm for 90° turns (750 mm for short obstructions)
Wheelchair turning circle	1500 mm	1500 mm	1500 mm
Specific rooms			
Living room	No minimum space standards	No minimum space standards. Must be at entrance level. Must allow a 1500 mm turning circle	No guidance
Kitchen	As for general housing but clear 1400 x 1400 mm for wheelchair manoeuvre	No minimum space standards Must allow a 1500 mm turning circle	No guidance
Dining space	No guidance	No minimum space standard Must allow a 1500 mm turning circle	No guidance
Bathroom/shower room	Wheelchair access not essential Room at same level as entrance to dwelling	No minimum space standard. Should allow wheelchair lateral transfer to WC and bath	No guidance

Table 6.2 continued

Housing design element	1974 HDDOP 2/74 Mobility Housing	1997 Lifetime Homes Standards	1999 The building Regulations Approved Document M: Access and Facilities for Disabled People
Specific rooms (cont'd)			
Toilet	No minimum space standards Same level as entrance	No minimum space standard. Ground floor with wheelchair access. Services for potential shower later	Entrance level WC 750 mm approach in front of WC Wheelchair access but not accommodation of wheelchair
Bedroom	No minimum space standards	No minimum space standards. Space identified for temporary bed space on ground floor	No guidance
Additional storage	No guidance	No guidance	No guidance
Other housing design elements			
Heating	Heating controls reachable by disabled person	No guidance on temperature. Fully automatic heating in Northern Ireland	No guidance
Egress in the event of fire	No guidance	No guidance	No guidance
Communication	No guidance	No guidance	No guidance
Position of controls	Align with door handles 1040 mm above floor level	600–1200 mm from finished floor level	450–1200 mm from finished floor level
Stairs	Standard staircase	Straight flight if possible Able to take stairlift later 900 mm minimum width of stairwell	Stairwell width 900 mm with continuous rail See approved Document Part K

general needs houses, flats and bungalows with relative ease and at little additional cost (Brewerton and Darton, 1997).

Lifetime homes are designed to meet the changing needs of a family throughout their lifetime, such as raising small children, accommodating a teenager with a broken leg, having grandparents to stay, promoting mobility for ambulant disabled people and visitability for wheelchair users. Consideration is also given to the changes of tenant, which may occur through the lifecycle of the home. As well as having inbuilt features which will help them meet the general needs of the population, they have also been designed to make them more cost-effective to adapt for people with more extensive needs. For example, stairwells can accept stairlifts, ceilings, tracking hoists and bathroom walls are suitable for grab rails and other fixtures. Although the term 'lifetime home' may give the impression that this house type is truly universal, in practice there are limitations as to how successfully they can be adapted for wheelchair users, particularly assisted wheelchair users (Brewerton and Darton, 1997).

While the house type can be adapted for an independent wheelchair user, this may involve a costly and time-consuming package of adaptations including:

* possible widening of the driveway;
* major redesign of the kitchen layout;
* provision of an inter-floor lift;
* creation of en suite bathroom/bedroom;
* potential modifications to the upstairs bathroom;
* installation of a shower facility either in the ground-floor WC area or upstairs bathroom;
* provision of grab rails.

If needs are known during a housing transfer, many wheelchair users may prefer to move directly into a wheelchair standard home to avoid disruptive adaptation work and delays.

Some of the limitations for assisted wheelchair users, which have been identified in subsequent research, include:

* limited wheelchair manoeuvring, approach and transfer space where inter-floor lifts are used in bedrooms particularly where a double bed is in situ (this assumes full occupancy of upstairs rooms where space cannot be found from adjoining bedrooms);
* compromised space for assisted showering where the ground-floor WC space has been adapted to include a shower facility; while the larger bathroom upstairs could be adapted, this would be expensive and it assumes that there is adequate space for an inter-floor lift (Blythe et al., 2002).

As a result it is recommended that a mix of lifetime homes and wheelchair standard housing are used in new-build housing schemes to meet the full spectrum of need in the population. This housing mix also helps to integrate disabled people into local communities.

Lifetime homes standards were formally published in 1997 by the Joseph Rowntree Foundation and were implemented in Northern Ireland in 1998 where they apply to new-build social housing. Lifetime homes standards were applied to registered social landlords in Wales in 2001. In England, the Greater London Authority has now accepted lifetime homes as the design standard for all new-build homes. For the first time lifetime homes standards will apply to new build privately owned as well as social housing in London. A 10 per cent quota of wheelchair standard housing or housing that is easily adaptable for wheelchair users will complement lifetime homes (Greater London Authority, 2004). This marks a significant development in advancing inclusive housing, and this model of applying lifetime homes across tenures may well be considered in other parts of the UK.

In Scotland, the standards in Housing for Varying Needs (Scotland, 1998) are used as a basis for funding new social housing.

Building regulations relating to access in domestic dwellings

The Department of the Environment has applied access standards for disabled people to public buildings in England and Wales since 1985. These regulations were revised in 1991 under part M of the regulations: Access and Facilities for Disabled People (Dodd, 1998). The 1991 regulations were again revised and extended for the first time to apply to domestic dwellings in England and Wales in 1999, with similar revisions in Northern Ireland and Scotland.

The application of building regulations regarding accessibility to domestic dwellings has been widely welcomed as it helps to promote social inclusion by making it easier for disabled people to visit people's homes, and they should gradually help to reduce the scale of future adaptations. Many of the standards including a ground-floor WC and general access provisions will be of considerable benefit for ambulant disabled people.

It should be remembered, however, that building regulations constitute minimal access standards and will not in themselves meet all the needs of everyday wheelchair users as:

- Topography or plot area can determine whether the approach to the entrance is level, ramped or stepped. If the approach to the dwelling is steep or limited in size, the standards can default to providing steps suitable for ambulant disabled people.
- There is no mandatory requirement to provide lifts to multi-storey flats or apartments.

- The WC space standards do not allow for the internal cubicle fully to contain a wheelchair with the door closed. This may result in an inability to close the toilet door independently after transfer with associated loss of privacy and dignity. There is insufficient space for assisted wheelchair transfer and the restricted space may actually make some transfers where there is minimal or no weight bearing in the lower limbs hazardous.
- The regulations do not set minimum space or design standards for all the rooms in the dwelling or, indeed, all the rooms on the ground floor (O'Brien, 1999).

This design gap between building regulations and the needs of disabled people has been formally recognised. In 1999 the Joseph Rowntree Foundation published *Meeting Part M and Designing Lifetime Homes,* in which a convincing case is made to design lifetime homes standards where possible in all tenures (Carroll et al., 1999). Further research evidence emerged from an evaluation of user benefits and an economic appraisal of lifetime homes in Northern Ireland (Blythe et al., 2002), which demonstrated the added benefits in terms of user satisfaction and economic benefits to enhance access standards for all housing from current building regulations to lifetime homes standards.

The Building Regulations Part M are currently undergoing further review by the ODPM. This review will consider enhancing the building regulations to incorporate lifetime homes standards (Habinteg Housing Association, 2005).

RNIB Cymru Housing Sight, 2003

This publication (Rees and Lewis, 2003) recommends a range of design standards for people with sight loss, an area in which there has been a relative deficit of design guidance applied to domestic housing (Awang, 2004). Many people who are ambulant or wheelchair users may also have some degree of sight loss, and, as many of these recommendations are low to medium cost if incorporated into new-build housing, it is recommended that they be given further consideration in all new-build housing.

The evolution of wheelchair standard housing

With reference to Table 6.3, this section identifies how wheelchair standard housing is evolving to become more inclusive over time. The standards described are primarily those used to advise new-build housing, although elements of the standards above have been utilised for housing adaptations. Three sets of design guidance have been selected, as they are influential standards for wheelchair housing and to illustrate an evolutionary process in action.

Table 6.3 Wheelchair standard housing, 1975–2004

Housing design element	1975 Wheelchair Standard Housing HDDOP 2/75	1997 NATWHAG Wheelchair Housing Design Guide	2001 BS: 8300 Design of buildings and their approaches to meet the needs of disabled people – code of practice
Access to dwellings	Gardens should be small	Useful new guidance on external elements	Extensive new guidance – see code of practice
Car parking	Where there is parking within curtilage (3400 mm wide) provide undercover access to the house	Covered hard standing. No spatial guidance identified. Rear car door entry identified	Firm level ground 3600 × 6000 mm markings for off-street parking spaces 4200 × 5700 mm for enclosed parking space
Paths	Not less than 1000 mm	1200 mm	1800 mm for buildings 1200 mm less busy routes 900 mm paths within curtilage of a single dwelling
Ramp/path gradient	1:20	1:20 1:12 up to 5000 mm length Level landing 1500 × 1500 mm	1:20 any steeper should conform to ramp specification 10 m – Max 1:20 5 m – Max 1:15 < 2 m – Max 1:12 ramp width 1200 Landing platform 1200 mm minimum
Main entrance/ threshold	Flush or near flush 15 mm upstand max	Covered entrance Upstand not to exceed 15 mm Additional weatherproofing details included	Canopy or recessed entrance Level or 15 mm upstand Chamfer upstand if more than 5 mm

Table 6.3 continued

Housing design element	1975 Wheelchair Standard Housing HDDOP 2/75	1997 NATWHAG Wheelchair Housing Design Guide	2001 BS: 8300 Design of buildings and their approaches to meet the needs of disabled people – code of practice
Lifts where applicable	Ground-floor provision preferred	BS5900 (1991) Shaft sizes: 1425 × 965 – 1190 × 785 mm	BS EN 81-1 BS EN 81-2 Internal dimensions: 1000 × 1250 mm wide one user of manual or electric chair. 1500 mm deep car will accommodate most scooters 1100 mm wide × 1400 mm deep one wheelchair user and companion 2000 mm wide × 1400 mm deep – a wheelchair user plus several other passengers in communal situations 1500 × 1500 mm manoeuvring space at approach
External doors Doorset Clear opening width	900–1000 mm 750 mm minimum	800 mm 300–550 mm clearance at lock edge on approach side	800 mm preferred 750 mm straight on access 850 mm if at right angles from 900 mm access route 300 mm clearance between leading edge of door and return wall
Internal doors Doorset Clear opening width	900 mm Assumes 775 mm	750–775 mm preferred	750 mm minimum straight on approach 800 mm preferred up to 800–850 mm preferred for 90° turn off 900 mm corridor
Door hanging	Sliding doors in certain circumstances	Wide variety of door types considered Preferable to open more than 90°	Wide variety of door types identified with separate guidance for each type Forces to operate door identified

Table 6.3 continued

Housing design element	1975 Wheelchair Standard Housing HDDOP 2/75	1997 NATWHAG Wheelchair Housing Design Guide	2001 BS: 8300 Design of buildings and their approaches to meet the needs of disabled people – code of practice
Corridors	1200 mm	900 mm for straight passage 1200 mm to allow 90° turn 1500 mm to allow 180° turn	Minimum clear width 900 mm for single family dwelling 1200 mm preferred. 1800 mm where there are two or more wheelchair users
Wheelchair turning space (T.C.)	1500 mm	1800 × 1400 mm	Wheelchair turning space variable 1500 × 1500 mm upwards
Living room	No minimum space standards	Rooms not narrower than 3000 mm wide. References to space for furniture and approach spaces	No minimum space standards This area was not commented on
Kitchen	Wheelchair TC 1500 mm – if there is any obstruction. 1400 mm between parallel surfaces if no obstructions	Wheelchair manoeuvring space 1800 mm × 1400 mm 400 mm between worktops	Unobstructed wheelchair manoeuvring 1500 × 1500 mm between facing floor units
Dining space	Space for 2 or 3 to sit down and eat in kitchen	No minimum space standards 1000 mm for approach space to table	No minimum standards Guidance on access to table
Bathroom/shower room	No minimum space standards – wheelchair accessible	No minimum dimensions identified 1000 × 1000 mm minimum level access shower space identified and 1500 or 1800 × 1400 mm turning space in the room identified	No single universal design identified 2700 × 3500 mm – assisted use 2700 × 2500 mm – independent use 2200 × 2000 mm – shower room independent user (no WC) 2500 × 2400 mm shower room with corner WC independent user 3100 × 2500 mm shower and WC for assisted independent user

Table 6.3 continued

Housing design element	1975 Wheelchair Standard Housing HDDOP 2/75	1997 NATWHAG Wheelchair Housing Design Guide	2001 BS: 8300 Design of buildings and their approaches to meet the needs of disabled people – code of practice
Toilet	1700 × 1400 mm or 1600 × 1500 mm 2 WCs in five-person dwelling	No minimum dimension identified 2 WCs preferred	1500 × 2200 mm Independent user 2200 × 2400 mm assisted wheelchair user – peninsular design
Bedroom	No minimum standards Examples given in design guide	No minimum space standards See guidance on layout of rooms Second bedroom desirable for visitors, carers, equipment	A sliding scale applies depending on bed and transfer space requirements Ranges from a single bedroom for an independent user 3900 × 3000 mm to a twin-bed arrangement for an assisted wheelchair user 3900 × 4850 mm
Additional storage	Storage guidance for kitchen 1200 × 700 mm. No location identified	See NHF Standards and Quality in Development: A Good Practice Guide. The value of having a spare bedroom was also identified for storage, as was the need for additional provision for specific equipment for wheelchair users	Total allowances in domestic dwellings not identified. General guidance to approach and layout of storage offered See also storage guidance for kitchen
Heating	22° in living/dining area 17° in other. Solid fuel not recommended	No specific temperature recommendations Even room temperatures recommended Low temperature radiator surfaces Controls within reach and usable	No specific guidance on air temperature Guidance on location of controls 750–1000 mm for heating controls requiring precise hand movement 41°C max temperature of heat emitters

Table 6.3 continued

Housing design element	1975 Wheelchair Standard Housing HDDOP 2/75	1997 NATWHAG Wheelchair Housing Design Guide	2001 BS: 8300 Design of buildings and their approaches to meet the needs of disabled people – code of practice
Egress in the event of fire	No comprehensive guidance	No specific guidance. Failsafe lighting and fire alarm recommended	Fire alarms should have both visual and audible signals
Communications	Telephone recommended	Multiple telephone sockets Can have emergency/alarm facilities Provide power supply for entry phone, door openers The need for specialist advice on environmental controls identified	Guidance on a range of communications equipment, e.g. entry phones, communications equipment for people with sensory impairment. Mostly applied to public buildings
Position of controls	Align with door handles	700–1000 mm 800 mm both sockets and switches Variances exist	Zones defined depending on nature of usage 750–1000 mm for controls requiring precise hand movements Meters between 1200 and 1400 mm from floor so people can reach and see them All outlets, switches and controls at least 350 mm from room corners
Additional spatial planning recommendations			A range of charts outlining space requirements for a range of wheelchair users is outlined
Clear passage between furniture		800 mm	
Clear space for side approach or use of facilities		1000 mm	1050 mm min
Space to approach furniture and reverse to pull out drawers		1350 mm	

HDOPP 2/75 Wheelchair Standard Housing 1975

This was developed by Goldsmith and Morton (1975) in response to the Chronically Sick and Disabled Persons Act 1970, which required local authorities to consider the housing needs of physically disabled people for the first time. This blueprint formed the baseline standards for much local authority new-build wheelchair housing from the 1970s to the 1990s.

The wheelchair users most carefully considered when developing these standards were independent self-propelling wheelchair users, who could often transfer independently and many of the spatial design standards were largely based on the performance and space requirements of the 8L manual self-propelling wheelchair (Goldsmith, 1963). These standards still largely meet the needs of independent wheelchair users.

It is now recognised that wheelchair users have considerably varying needs. There is a greater range of wheelchairs on the market with varying manoeuvring and performance characteristics. Assisted wheelchair users and their carers have additional spatial needs, which need to be considered (O'Brien, 1999).

National Wheelchair Housing Association Group (NATWHAG):
Wheelchair Housing Design Guide (1997)

This guide based on in-depth research with twenty wheelchair users (occupational therapists were involved in ten of the studies) was to establish guidance for new-build wheelchair standard housing in England. It also influenced the Housing Corporation Scheme Development Standards, which are used to determine funding for new social housing.

This publication identified new guidance in a number of areas, including:

1. design guidance on external elements such as moving around outside and using outdoor spaces;
2. consideration of additional space to accommodate wheelchair access to rear-entry vehicles;
3. a more generous turning circle allowance (1800 × 1400 mm) applied to living room, kitchen and bathrooms/shower rooms;
4. a minimum space standard for living rooms;
5. the desirability of a second bedroom for visitors, carers and equipment;
6. improved standards for the provision of facilities to support the installation of communications equipment in the home;
7. additional spatial planning guidance regarding use of furniture.

The British Standards Institute BS: 8300 Design of Buildings and Their
Approaches to Meet the Needs of Disabled People (2001)

The recommendation for this study originated from the Department for the Environment and the Regions' studies in 1997 and 2001 respectively. PD 6523 cited in BSI, 2001 p. v:

concluded that that the guidance with respect to the access needs of disabled people was incomplete, in some instances contradictory and on the whole not based on validated research.

This code of practice has received much attention as it was underpinned by a substantial ergonomic study of the needs of wheelchair users and is considered to form best practice.

Indeed, there has been discussion as to whether it should form the 'deemed to satisfy' benchmark for the Disability Discrimination Act 1995 in public buildings.

Although BS: 8300 offers guidance on good practice in the design of both domestic and non-domestic buildings and their approaches, it requires considerable interpretation to apply design elements to domestic dwellings. The researchers recognised that there may be a requirement for future dwelling-specific guidance. To date, these standards have not been generally applied to domestic new-build wheelchair standard housing, although they are considered in the Greenwich wheelchair site brief (Greenwich Council, 2002). They have influenced some recently published housing adaptations design guidance (NIHE, 2004).

In an attempt to get some sense of how the application of BS: 8300 may impact on the design of future wheelchair standard housing, some key design elements have been identified and compared with previous standards in the chart.

The central developments are:

1. considerably strengthened guidance on the approaches to buildings;
2. increased space standards for car parking and valuable spatial guidance on a range of vehicle approach scenarios;
3. enhanced guidance on the design of entrance door thresholds;
4. comprehensive guidance on a variety of lift options;
5. flexible guidance on door/corridor width relationships;
6. a range of options for utilising varying door types;
7. considerably increased space standards for assisted wheelchair users in bathroom/shower rooms and toilets;
8. enhanced design guidance on the design of bedrooms particularly for assisted wheelchair users;
9. specific guidance on the location of controls relating to functional requirements;
10. comprehensive data from user trials to inform reach ranges and general space requirements.

This source of design guidance at least partially addresses the deficit of design guidance in earlier publications for assisted wheelchair users and carers in the locations where carers offer personal assistance, i.e. bathrooms, toilets and bedrooms (living rooms were not considered). Guidance on space for carers to assist and use mobile hoists is outlined, although the space savings achievable through the use of fixed-track ceiling hoists were not examined.

Although 1500 mm has been identified in the main text of BS: 8300 as the turning space allowance for the main living areas, when appendix E is explored in detail it becomes apparent that the actual space requirements to turn through 180° are much larger.

Eighty per cent of self-propelled and electrically propelled wheelchair users required a length of 2000 mm and a width of 1500 mm to turn. A full 360° turn or circle would take more space again. This is a significant finding and may well have quite considerable implications for spatial planning in wheelchair standard dwellings.

General wheelchair housing trends

There is evidence that as wheelchair standards develop they are becoming more inclusive for a wider range of wheelchair users. The original blueprint by Goldsmith gave greatest emphasis to the needs of independent wheelchair users but as time has progressed the needs of wheelchair users with more complex needs are being addressed. By 2001 assisted wheelchair users and carers are formally considered in BS: 8300 and now Rees and Lewis (2003), where consideration is given to people with sight loss. As more inclusive design standards have emerged, there has also been a gradual increase in the overall space allowances for wheelchair standard housing and improvements in the design of the approaches and car parking.

Further research and development work on wheelchair housing will be required to address:

- egress in the event of a fire;
- control of home heating;
- enhancing personal security in the home;
- improving storage solutions;
- home automation/environmental controls;
- minimum space standards in various rooms;
- improved flooring;
- design for sensory loss;
- low maintenance and accessible gardens.

A more inclusive design approach to new-build wheelchair standard housing has the potential to reduce the need for expensive and time-consuming adaptations and to maximise the potential for relets.

Conclusion

As one examines the historical trends which are improving accessibility in housing, it is possible to observe a gradual application of building regulations and access standards from public buildings over to domestic dwellings, starting with social housing and finally moving into privately owned property.

We have seen step-by-step improvements in access standards applied to housing in the UK, with building regulations tending to lag behind best practice emerging from research and development. The reason for this time lag primarily comes from opposition from the building industry to enhanced space standards, which may reduce immediate profit margins. A truly holistic cost-benefit analysis of providing more inclusive new-build housing needs to be undertaken, measuring the real health and social benefits of this provision such as: independence, social integration, reduction in home accidents, disease prevention from improved heating, reduced expenditure on home/residential care, earlier hospital discharge and the reduction of adaptations expenditure (Blythe et al., 2002; Cobbold, 1997).

If a full analysis of benefits is undertaken, society as a whole might conclude that the creation of inclusive housing is indeed 'money well spent' (Heywood, 2001).

Key points

- The history of inclusive design in the built environment is a relatively short one, emerging in the 1960s. In just over forty years this area has seen major advances in the design of public buildings followed by domestic dwellings, first in social housing and more recently in new-build privately owned property.
- Within the OT focus on occupational performance, a number of models offer the practitioner a philosophical rationale for developing a deeper understanding of the person–environment interface.
- Universal design, which originated in the USA, is having a major impact on societies' approaches to the design of everyday products and the built environment. It promotes equality of opportunity and an inclusive design process.
- User-centred design also offers practitioners an evidence-based approach to the evaluation and development of inclusive design standards.
- Mobility housing, conceptualised by Selwyn Goldsmith, was the first major attempt to have a 'mainstream' or general needs house type, which would also be suitable for disabled people.

- Lifetime homes have further developed the concept of mainstream housing to meet changing needs through a family's lifecycle and have also incorporated features to make housing easier to adapt. There are practical constraints to the adaptation of lifetime homes for assisted wheelchair users.
- There are varying definitions of wheelchair standard housing. Further research and development work is required to create inclusive design solutions, which meet the needs of assisted wheelchair users and their carers.

Acknowledgements

The author would like to thank the following people for their guidance and support in this chapter:

Adrian Blythe, Design Support Service Manager, Northern Ireland Housing Executive.

Mike Woods, Strategy and Development Manager, Housing and Technical Resources, South Lanarkshire Council.

Trevor Dodd and Beth Atkinson, Housing Senior Occupational Therapists, Housing Disability Team, Greenwich Council.

CHAPTER 7

Housing adaptations and community care

CLARE PICKING

This chapter considers the role of occupational therapists working within UK local authority settings in arranging home adaptations for disabled people and looks at how these services can best be provided within the context of community care services. The chapter considers the need to balance the importance of understanding the legal background and various funding routes for adaptations while making individualised recommendations which meet users' needs and follow professional standards.

There is strong emphasis on partnership with disabled people and their carers in taking decisions about changes to the home and between housing and social care services in agreeing and carrying out the work. A creative approach is adopted to both empower users and ensure that professional colleagues recognise the role of occupational therapists as crucial, rather than marginal, within community care.

Introduction

Occupational therapists working in local authorities play a central role in providing community care services when recommending housing adaptations which enable independent living. Increasing numbers of NHS occupational therapists find themselves working in community settings, extending their own roles further into the home and integrating more closely with their local authority colleagues. They contribute to the housing adaptation role and must also appreciate a clear understanding of the statutory perspectives, the dilemmas and, in some cases, inconsistencies of adaptation work.

The chapter sets the occupational therapist role within its legal context and covers funding options for community care services specifically in England, since these aspects vary in approach in other parts of the UK. Those parts of the chapter which cover the main professional issues of assessment, planning interventions with users and translating needs into adaptations can, however, be seen in a wider, more global context.

Adaptations in community care

What are community care services?

Community care services are set out in s 47 of the NHS and Community Care (NHS&CC) Act 1990 together with those that are covered in s 2 of the Chronically Sick and Disabled Persons (CSDP) Act 1970 (hereafter referred to as community care legislation). They generally assist people to remain living in their own homes and include practical help, equipment and 'assistance with home adaptations and/or additional facilities for greater safety, comfort and convenience' (CSDP Act 1970, s 2).

With a legal commitment to enable disabled people to live as independently as they wish in the community and with an increasingly ageing population, it has become necessary for local authorities to develop a broad approach to care in the community, providing an alternative to residential care. In 1990 the NHS&CC Act introduced the concept of a needs-led rather than a service-led approach, emphasising the importance of independent living. The key themes were:

- to enable individuals to live as normal a life as possible in their own homes or in a homely environment in the community;
- to provide sufficient care and support to help people to achieve maximum independence and, by acquiring or re-acquiring basic living skills, to help them achieve their full potential as individuals;
- to give people a voice in how they live their lives and what services they need.

Community care services cover a range of options for individuals to continue living in their own homes, which together form a 'package of care'. The options can include practical support in the home, day care, equipment, adaptations, delivery of meals, transport and so on. The services can be arranged by council professionals and are provided by a variety of different agencies.

The care management approach

Under community care legislation, local authority social care services are the lead agencies for assessing and arranging community care services as enablers and purchasers, rather than main providers, using a process called care management. Care management involves different levels and types of assessments, proportionate to the presenting need, by council staff including 'care managers', who might have a range of professional backgrounds including social work, home care, nursing or occupational therapy. This approach ensures that:

- an assessment of need is carried out either by care managers or other appropriate professionally or vocationally qualified persons and that assessments are proportionate to the level of need;
- an individual care plan is devised with the service user's agreement;
- the level of eligible need is decided upon, with reference to the local authority's eligibility criteria;
- co-ordination of services occurs using the statutory or independent sectors;
- services are monitored and reviewed regularly.

Occupational therapists sometimes co-ordinate care packages as part of their role or, more usually, contribute to the process by providing a specialist assessment, which might be simple or complex. They may work jointly with care managers or work alone and arrange certain community care services to contribute to a care package, which may include equipment and adaptations.

The Single (or Unified) Assessment Process

The Single Assessment Process forms part of the care management process and arises from the National Service Framework for Older People to assist in simplifying health and social care assessments by keeping them in proportion to needs. Every agency contributes to the assessment process, using a common assessment tool and a shared IT system to encourage communication and avoid duplication. Occupational therapists are expected to contribute to this process, particularly with specialist and comprehensive assessments.

The relationship between housing and community care

Housing services are a core component of community care; suitable housing is not only an integral part of the shift from residential to community-based care but also provides a stable base for independent living and affords access to other services such as health and social care, education and training (Audit Commission, 1998).

Since the intention behind care in the community was to reduce the numbers of people using residential facilities and transfer their care to a local setting, inevitably the housing requirements of community-based care have changed:

- Increasing numbers of people with high care needs, including those receiving palliative or continuing health care, can choose to be cared for in the community rather than in hospitals or hospices.
- Recognition that people might have a combination of impairments and that families can have more than one member who is disabled. This can occur particularly when large extended families live together, including in the ethnic minority population.
- Changes in funding arrangements, such as the Direct Payments Act (Great Britian 1996b), offering a wider range of living options.
- The Manual Handling Regulations (1992), which have led to more space requirements for (hoisting) equipment and carer activity.
- Availability of a developing and versatile range of equipment for daily living and wheelchairs.

The implications of changed requirements in the home are that more space is required, for example for specialist furniture or medical equipment and for care provision. Many of these changes have to be addressed by adaptations as, unless it has been built to new regulations, existing housing is rarely suitable for disabled people.

The need for adaptations

Internal and external environmental barriers are not apparent until the resident is challenged by impairment; steps and stairs, changes in levels, the design of baths, narrow doorways and confined WC areas all present potential difficulties. Although moving to a more suitable home is an option, it is more likely that an adaptation will be the preferred option to meet individual need.

Adaptations which give access throughout the home are likely to maintain or increase mobility and independence which in turn influence general good health or prevent further deterioration through immobility. Research by Heywood (2001) shows that 77 per cent of respondents felt that their adaptation, including the benefits of adequate heating, had produced a good health outcome. Heywood (2004) also indicates that well-designed adaptations have beneficial or even preventative effects on both physical and mental health and help other family members. In particular disabled people reported pain, depression and fear of accidents and care-givers reported back injuries, falls and stress before an adaptation was carried out.

Home adaptations are divided into two main types, minor adaptations and major adaptations.

Minor adaptations

These adaptations are usually classified as such if they cost below approximately £1000. They are usually funded through social care budgets and are therefore, as for equipment, considered to be community care services. They include grab rails or rails for stairs and outside steps, small ramps, door widening and so on. They are used as the initial solution in most instances in order to maintain function at home and to minimise risk. Very often these adaptations, if promptly fitted, can help a person remain at home (Mountain, 2000), avoid a hospital admission, assist the carer and reduce or remove the necessity for a care package.

Minor adaptations can minimise risk and reduce care packages.
• A rail by the bath and bathing equipment may provide independence in personal hygiene and remove the need for assistance.
• An extra rail on the stairs might remove the need for a bed and commode in a downstairs living room and a care worker to empty the commode.
• Re-hanging a bedroom door might allow space for a person with a walking frame to manage getting up and dressed without a care worker to assist.

Major adaptations

Wherever possible, these adaptations, usually costing more than the £1000 financial cut-off, will be achieved by keeping within the existing structure of the home, since more extensive work is both costly and disruptive.

Occupational therapists assess for and authorise major adaptations, which are funded outside their own social care budgets, by the Disabled Facilities Grant (DFG) system, council housing or housing association budgets. These adaptations are not strictly called community care services, despite their importance in enabling care in the community, simply because they are funded by different providers.

Since occupational therapists play such a large role in recommending adaptations for the home setting, it is important to examine that role in more detail.

The occupational therapist's housing role in the community

Once it is clear that rehabilitation or equipment are not appropriate, the occupational therapist combines the assessment of the individual and their home environment with the translation of identified needs into a variety of solutions including home adaptations. The enabling role of the occupational therapist assists the decision-making, and it is the appreciation of the limiting effect of the environment upon people with impairment, the very essence of the social model of disability (see Chapter 3), which places the occupational therapist in an ideal position to maximise the potential of the home environment.

The occupational therapist has been described as the key player in bringing housing issues into a community care assessment (Joseph Rowntree Foundation, 1998). Increasingly, this function is provided not only by occupational therapists in social care services but also by those in NHS and housing authority settings. Franklin (1998) describes how the occupational therapist's integrated and person-centred approach displays a full grasp of the inter-dependency between person and home, home and person. The link between the impairment of the individual and the constraints placed upon their ability to function by the immediate environment forms the main area of expertise and intervention.

Creek describes how:

> analysis of the environment may provide information about the causes of problems for the individual, explanations for behaviour or ideas for therapeutic modifications. Environmental analysis includes:
>
> • Objective observation and recording of who and what is there (content analysis).
> • Appraisal of the effects of the environment on people and their perceptions, behaviours and participation in occupations and activities (demand analysis).
> • Identification of elements which need to be altered and the means by which this may be one (adaptive analysis). (Creek, 2003, p. 38)

Creek also lists environmental adaptation among the core skills of an occupational therapist in:

> making temporary or permanent changes to the client's physical, cultural, institutional or social environments in order to influence her/his level of motivation and/or facilitate occupational performance. Occupation shapes, and is shaped by, space therefore changes in any aspects of the environment will affect occupation and occupational performance. The therapist needs to appreciate how existing spaces are perceived and used before recommending any adaptation. (ibid)

The COT wishes to see health and social care models of occupational therapy combining in the future into a (specialist) general occupational therapy practitioner role. This role will provide rehabilitation/treatment services, a sound range of disability equipment (assistive technologies) and basic housing adaptations (COT, 2002, section 3.14). Many NHS occupational therapists are already carrying out these functions, often working closely with their social care colleagues.

Occupational therapists in housing departments advise on adapting existing homes and can be involved in the selection of more suitable alternatives, grading void (empty) properties, assisting in compiling housing property registers to ensure suitable lettings and advising on refurbishment or new-build schemes. They may assess individual need, including homeless people, before a home is offered and inspect any potentially suitable void properties. The offer of a home and possible adaptations to it should link with any care package that might be arranged.

The occupational therapist role in both social care and the wider housing setting is influenced by a complex agenda of legislation which provides a strong framework for practice, unlike its counterpart in the NHS. The following section covers the basics of this framework and demonstrates not only some of the inconsistencies but also how recent changes have assisted the occupational therapist to work in a more holistic way.

The legal background

One important difference between health, social care and housing services is that, whereas health services are not generally governed by legislation, all social care services (community care) must be assessed for and provided under specific legislation, as with housing services.

Social care services

There is a statutory requirement (a duty) under s 47 of the NHS&CC Act for local social care services to assess anyone who 'appears to be in need of community care services'. This requirement to assess will be fulfilled by various social care staff dependent on the particular presenting need. Occupational therapists mainly assess disabled and older people under two Acts (the CSDP Act 1970 and the Disabled Persons Act 1986). It is usually sufficient to know that a person has a 'permanent and substantial' disability and could therefore be 'registered' or 'registerable' under the CSDP Act for the duty to assess to be triggered. Disability is defined under s 29 of the National Assistance Act 1948. Children are eligible for an assessment of their needs and assistance if they are 'in need' under the Children Act 1989. Services must 'minimize the effect (of disability) on disabled children . . . and give them the opportunity to lead lives which are as normal as possible'.

Although NHS occupational therapists in community settings have not in the past assessed for or provided equipment or adaptations for their patients under any specific legislation, where their recommendations are funded by local authorities they must adhere to the local social care eligibility criteria, clinical reasoning and policies. The Health Acts 1977 and 1999 also allow for co-operation and partnership between health and local authorities to pool resources to provide joint services in the prevention and aftercare of people suffering with illness.

All decisions for the provision of community care services following assessments are based on Fair Access to Care Services (FACS) Guidance (DOH, 2002a). This is statutory guidance based upon care management guidance (DOH/SSI, 1991), the results of Ombudsman enquiries and interpretive court decisions. FACS provides social care services with a framework for a consistent approach to eligibility for services. Assessments, including those by occupational therapists, are used to determine 'eligible' need for community care services. Local authorities must set a low threshold to avoid screening individuals out of the assessment process before sufficient information is known about them. The eligibility framework has four bands (critical, substantial, moderate and low) which refer to 'the seriousness of the risk to a person's independence or other consequences if needs are not addressed' (DOH, 2002a, 13, s 16). There are four categories (s 40) which should be given equal weight in determining eligible need:

- autonomy and freedom to make choices;
- health and safety including freedom from harm, abuse and neglect, and taking wider issues of housing and community safety into account;
- the ability to manage personal and other daily routines;
- involvement in family and wider community life, including leisure, hobbies, unpaid and paid work, learning and volunteering.

The word vital as used in the context of the critical band of the eligibility framework means that without help individuals are at great risk of either losing their independence, possibly necessitating admission to institutional care or making very little, damaging or inappropriate contributions to family or wider community life with serious consequences for the individual and others.

The implications of FACS for occupational therapists are that there is considerable scope to ensure holistic needs are met within a broad framework. However, people who do not meet the local eligibility criteria might still have disability-related housing needs, which would be funded either by the various housing budgets or DFG. The occupational therapy role here, after assessment, might be that of making a recommendation for adaptations and helping to re-route the disabled person to another agency.

Table 7.1 The eligibility framework banding

Band	Description	Example of how this might apply
Critical	The service user has either life-threatening unmet needs or a failure to meet their needs will lead to vital consequences within the four categories of need	The service user relies (or would need to rely) upon assistance at all times of the day, cannot reach any essential facilities safely or independently and would not be able to manage living in their home environment without suitable support
Substantial	If the assessed needs are not met, the majority of the service user's support systems will be at risk	The service user relies (or would need to rely) upon assistance several times a day, cannot reach most essential facilities safely or independently and would have great difficulty living in their home environment and managing their lifestyle without suitable support
Moderate	If the assessed needs are not met, several of the service user's support systems will be at risk	The service user relies (or would need to rely) upon some assistance during the day or week, can reach some but not all essential facilities safely and independently and would have some difficulty living in their home environment and managing their lifestyle without suitable support
Low	If the assessed needs are not met, some (one or two) of the service user's support systems will be at risk	The service user does not usually rely (or would not need to rely) upon assistance during the day or the week, can reach most but not all essential facilities safely and independently but might have some difficulty living in their home environment and managing their lifestyle without suitable support

Housing services

The Local Government and Housing Act 1989 (Great Britian, 1989b) intro-duced DFGs providing both mandatory and discretionary funding for housing adaptations. The scope of these grants was extended by the Housing Grants Construction and Regeneration Act 1996 (Great Britian, 1996a), which also extended the definition of disability. DFGs cannot be restricted by a local authority's lack of resources but are means tested and subject to a financial ceiling. In contrast to the system for the allocation of community care servic-es, there are no resource-limited eligibility criteria to meet in the context of housing services. The 1989 Housing Act requires social service departments (usually occupational therapists) to assess whether the adaptations they rec-ommend are 'necessary and appropriate' in order to fund DFGs.

The Regulatory Reform Order (2002) introduced changes to private sector housing grants and abolished discretionary grants. More flexibility was given to local authorities in deciding how to assist applicants with discretionary payments, and options can include equity release, assistance in moving home and use of small grants to fund fast-track adaptations.

Occupational therapy interventions in the social care setting are tightly governed by legislation and guidance and underpinned by strong professional expertise in assessments making recommendations as part of a care plan leading to problem-solving and decision-making, which will be considered in the following sections.

Occupational therapy assessment and planning

Assessment

The simple or proportionate assessments described in the care management process are sometimes quite different from the assessment for which an occupational therapist is trained. The holistic approach to the disabled person taken by the occupational therapist involves the assessment of the home environment, leisure, work, educational and social needs together with physical, cognitive and psychological factors.

FACS guidance encourages flexibility in these areas, the use of preventative measures and the need to explore the intensity of particular needs including the physical pain, distress or disruption they cause. Guidance (ODPM, 2004) assists the assessment process in connection with adaptations, placing emphasis on a partnership approach with disabled people and their carers.

The Single Assessment Process for older people, to which the occupational therapist must contribute, provides guidance on assessment scales and indicates the domains of the process that must be covered. Many of these scales will resonate with an occupational therapist as they include personal care, physical well-being, the immediate environment and resources.

The more complex occupational therapist assessment in relation to housing combines measurement of individual functional status in activities of daily living (ADL) with an analysis of the environment and the abilities of the carer. Many of the formal functional status measuring tools are unsuited to local authority work, either because they do not include domestic activities, are insensitive to the outcomes of equipment or adaptations or have not been validated for use in the community (Heaton and Bamford, 2001).

However, in a study of the effectiveness of the local authority provision for children, which included major and minor adaptations, Stewart and Neyerlin-Beale (2000) found that both the Canadian Occupational

Performance Measure (Law et al., 1994) and the Community Dependency Index (Eakin and Baird, 1995) were relevant assessment tools. Iwarsson (1999) developed an objective tool in Sweden for assessing accessibility in the housing and immediate outdoor environment, but this has yet to be validated for the UK. Clemson et al. (1999) considered the content validity of the Westmead Safety Assessment Tool (Clemson et al. 1992; Clemson, 1997) in identifying home fall hazards and conclude that it is a potential guide if used together with therapists' knowledge and expertise.

Risk assessment

Assessment of risk plays a substantial part in the work of an occupational therapist. It has traditionally been associated with moving and handling assessments (see Chapter 8), but in fact extends to every area of life at home. For instance, the therapist must weigh up the inherent risk involved in making any recommendation which might extend or enable an activity in the home and reduce the care package but increase risk in other ways.

Case study 7.1: example of a risk assessment relating to a stairlift
An elderly person sleeps downstairs in the living room and manages most ADLs with support from formal carers. The installation of a stairlift would give the person full use of their home with a reduction of the care package, but their condition includes bouts of giddiness, poor balance and is deteriorating, with a possible increase in risk (of falling) were the stairlift to be fitted. The risk to safety might therefore be greater than the need to give full access around the home.

Assessing the risk of falling is particularly important in planning home adaptations for older people. In an international review of the literature on falls, Lord et al. (2001) observe that environmental risk does play a part in causing falls. When carrying out ordinary tasks and if more than one environmental factor is present, older, more vigorous people are more likely to fall than the frail older person, who is likely to fall regardless of environmental factors. People with particular disabilities such as stroke or amputation and cognitive impairments are also more vulnerable in this way. They comment that the relationship between environmental factors and the extent of injury indicates that falls on stairs double the risk of serious injury.

Government guidance (National Institute for Clinical Excellence, 2004) makes clear the importance of home hazard assessment and safety intervention/modifications following hospital discharge after a fall but makes clear that this is only effective in conjunction with follow-up and intervention.

Disabled people should be encouraged to manage their own needs and risks in partnership with the therapist, who must balance the right of the mentally competent adult to autonomy, with the duty of care owed by the healthcare professional to the client. The therapist must take into account foreseeable risks, what reasonable action should be taken to meet those risks and that it is 'in accordance with the reasonable standards of professional practice' (Dimond, 1997, p. 317). The disabled person should be made aware of any risks they might be taking when planning to continue living alone, for example, or allowing their informal carer to continue to provide care rather than accept outside help or equipment.

Assessment of carers

Under the Carers (Recognition and Services) Act 1995 (Great Britian 1995a), any carer who is providing or intends to provide care on a regular basis has the right to an assessment of their ability to care or continue to care and that assessment should be taken into account when determining the services to be provided. The needs of carers from minority ethnic groups must also be considered within the context of family and cultural traditions.

Where the cared-for person is eligible for community care services but refuses to accept these services, for instance equipment or an adaptation, the carer may be assessed under the Carers and Disabled Children Act 2000, and the local authority then has the discretion to provide the carer with a range of supportive services to assist their caring role, although they are not obliged to do so.

The completion of the assessment process is achieved once the occupational therapist feels that all aspects of the presenting difficulties have been explored and understood and have been placed into the context of need. Needs must then be addressed, but solutions might not be apparent at this stage.

Preparing an intervention (care) plan

Once the needs have been identified, the next stage in the care management process is to prepare a care plan with the disabled person or, for an occupational therapist, possibly more appropriately called an intervention plan, which is not to be confused with the professional assessment report. In establishing needs the occupational therapist listens carefully to the disabled person and takes their views into account. Although a particular difficulty may seem to be a priority to the assessor, it may not be a high priority for the individual, who may attach more importance to another area of their life altogether. The purpose of this careful exploration of need is to reach an agreement on what will later be required to meet their needs.

It is important to consult carers or specialist advisers to ensure all aspects of the person's life have been taken into account. Any decision made, when part of an overall care plan, must be shared with a care manager or other professionals involved, to encourage a joint approach to the future support or otherwise of the individual. Setting objectives rather than looking at funding at this stage can assist with intervention planning.

Case study 7.2: setting objectives for an intervention plan
Mrs A is of working age. She lives in her own home and uses a wheelchair. She would like to go out to work and do her own shopping and cooking but has no level access into or within her home. There are two steps at the front door, the kitchen door is very narrow and the units are standard and the bathroom and WC are very small with standard fittings. She has difficulty washing herself all over, in sitting up from lying down in bed and sitting at her dining table to eat meals since the table is too high. Her eligible needs fall into the substantial band of the local eligibility criteria.
A summary of Mrs A's needs might be:

- to have access in and out of the house to allow her to return to work and do her own shopping;
- to have access to washing, toileting and cooking facilities in her home;
- to maintain personal hygiene independently;
- to sit up in bed independently;
- to eat meals at a suitable height surface in her wheelchair.

Once the needs have been identified, the intervention plan is a crucial tool for identifying how need is to be met and by whom. Needs may be met by:

- the local authority if they (the needs) meet their eligibility criteria;
- by the housing authority or grants department (for adaptations);
- by the voluntary sector (for example a bathing service or a small grant for furniture);
- the disabled person or their family.

Case study 7.2: Planning how objectives will be achieved
Decisions about who will meet Mrs A's needs are based on:

- type of housing tenure for the adaptations and/or
- her eligibility for local authority or other statutory services.

Stating the need may or may not be accompanied by a detailed solution. At this stage the therapist has only stated that Mrs A needs to have wheelchair access into and within the home at the front door, the bathroom and kitchen, not *how* it is to be achieved as this may not yet be decided (e.g. ramp, widening doors, shower, step lift etc.). If Mrs A's assessed needs fall below the local authority eligibility criteria threshold, then the third column (see below) will contain details of alternative suggested ways of meeting her need, such as for changing the table and leasing the car.

Note that any needs connected with her wish to return to work will be viewed with equal importance as her personal care needs under FACS guidance.

If the scope of the DFG does not cover any of the proposals because it would be considered discretionary and not mandatory, then the social care services would be required to fund it because her needs in this case fall within their eligibility criteria. More detailed solutions and specifications to the expressed needs for equipment and adaptations follow once the therapist has decided who is to meet the need and involved that agency in the planning.

Table 7.2 An example of an intervention plan which might be used by an occupational therapist

Type of need	How to be met (recommendation)	By whom
To have access in and out of her house to enable her to return to work and do her own shopping	By installation of level access at the front door for a wheelchair	Disabled Facilities Grant
	Transport by car	Mrs A to lease a car using Disabled Living Allowance
To have access to washing, toileting and cooking facilities	By internal adaptation to her home, giving wheelchair access to and within the bathroom and kitchen	Disabled Facilities Grant
To maintain personal hygiene independently	By installation of accessible washing facilities	Disabled Facilities Grant
To sit up in bed independently	By use of equipment – a pillow lifter	Social care services
To eat meals at a suitable height surface in her wheelchair	By use of a lower table	Private purchase or charity grant (furniture not provided by statutory funding)

Partnership working

Social care occupational therapists work with health colleagues, housing authorities, Home Improvement Agencies and grants officers in order to assist the disabled person through the complex adaptation process. They must also work in partnership with care managers as the successful outcome of an adaptation can have other further-reaching implications. These can include reducing (in cost) a care package (Mountain, 2000, p. 20) avoiding admission to hospital or residential place and speeding up hospital discharge.

Case study 7.3: use of adaptations to reduce a care package
Mrs S has recently returned home after a hospital admission following a fall and fractured neck of femur. She has osteoarthritis of both knees and a heart condition and is anxious about using the stairs to reach her bedroom and bathroom. A bed has been placed in the back living room with a commode nearby, and a care package has been arranged for three times a day to help her get up, wash and dress using a bowl on the kitchen table, to empty the commode, prepare meals and snacks and help her get ready for bed at night.

Mrs S is now becoming more confident in her transfers, is dressing herself and preparing drinks and meals, but will continue to need help with the commode and maintaining personal hygiene. A risk assessment shows that it would not be safe for her to use the stairs alone in the future to reach the WC.

The care manager may be considering a lengthy care package or a residential placement at any stage of this process and needs to know if an adaptation could be considered. Whether it is to install a stairlift or a shower/WC cubicle in the back living room, Mrs S might become independent in washing and toileting and, with no commode to empty, this may then reduce or remove altogether the need for a care package.

In some circumstances, working closely might resolve a potentially difficult situation.

Case study 7.4: a joint approach to ensure the right adaptation is provided
Mrs T has had a mild stroke and is finding it difficult to bath independently. She has been treated for depression for a long time and is threatening to self-harm if she is not provided with a shower. Her family gives a lot of support and she attends a day centre once a week, but refuses to attend more frequently. She has assistance to wash herself at home three times a week from a carer and from her family at weekends.

Following a joint assessment between the social care and specialist mental health occupational therapists and the care manager a decision is made to fit a level-access shower funded by a small grant from the local council grants department under their discretionary funding arrangements.

The decision to treat this request more quickly takes into account the FACS banding she would come under – the risks to her independence were the adaptation not to be provided and the need to avoid the lengthy DFG process. Once she appreciates that her needs are being understood, Mrs S agrees to attend the centre three times a week and have a shower there as a temporary measure.

An occupational therapist can also turn to the care manager to assist with funding an adaptation if a solution can be found which costs less than a temporary nursing home bed (see next section on alternative funding options on p. 156).

Funding adaptations

Funding adaptations is determined by the type of housing tenure and is administered either by social care services, the relevant housing authority or the grants department The range of options and restrictions in funding and the overlap in legislation, often encouraging variations in interpretation within and between authorities, can pose dilemmas for the occupational therapist in assisting disabled people in achieving their wishes. Figure 7.1 illustrates the various funding routes.

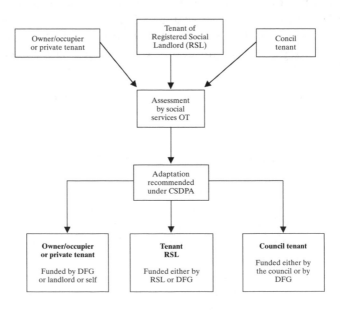

Figure 7.1 The funding routes of adaptations.

Owner/occupiers and private tenants

DFGs provide the main funding for adaptations and are available to any person irrespective of housing tenure; they are means tested and the applicant may be required to make a contribution based on the concept of an 'affordable loan', calculated on income and savings, but not on out-goings. The contribution is not based on the cost of the work involved and sometimes, if the applicant has considerable savings or income, it is larger than the expected costs, which leads applicants to withdraw from the process and fund the work privately. This is particularly the case with parents of disabled children.

DFGs are administered by grants officers based in local authorities and working closely with occupational therapists. Departmental resources are not taken into account when awarding grants, but there is a financial grant ceiling of £25,000 in England. Large-scale adaptations often cost much more than this ceiling, and any additional funding must be met either by the applicant or the local authority if the person's needs fall within the local eligibility criteria.

Council tenants

Funding for adaptations to council housing is complex and varied. They may be funded either by the local housing department or by DFG; councils sometimes waive the means test for applicants, while others apply it. Adaptations to council housing that has been transferred to housing trusts under Large Scale Voluntary Transfer must be funded by the trust unless the transfer took place in the early stages of the scheme, when a DFG might then be used. Within any two-tier council (a county council and district or borough councils), a combination of these arrangements is likely to exist.

Tenants of RSLs (housing associations or housing trusts)

The Housing Corporation as the parent body has no statutory responsibility to fund adaptations but has traditionally done so. It provides a Social Housing Grant to fund adaptations if the RSL has a substantial amount in their revenue budget. Often, however, the RSL uses the DFG system, unless (as described above), there has been a transfer of housing stock and an undertaking to fund adaptations.

Social care financial responsibilities and dilemmas for the occupational therapist

The occupational therapist must use the local funding routes, but responsibility for funding adaptations ultimately lies with social care services if funding is not forthcoming and the person meets their eligibility criteria. If, for instance, a grants department refuses to approve a DFG application, because the needs do not fall within the scope of a mandatory grant, or an RSL refuses to fund an adaptation, then the duty to assist defaults to social care services.

There are certain situations which pose a dilemma for the occupational therapist, where funding and type of housing tenure might represent a lack of equity and influence the recommendation.

Case study 7.5: differences in provision tied to resources and types of housing tenure

Miss B has needs which fall below the social care services eligibility threshold. She would benefit from rails and equipment in her bathroom and these cannot be provided by the social care services.

- *If she lives in her own or a privately rented home*, then no rails can be fitted (as stated above) and she would have to buy her own equipment.
- *If she lives in a council-owned home or an RSL-owned home*, then a grab rail might be fitted but she would have to buy her own equipment.

She might, however, be eligible for an adaptation funded by a DFG, which has different criteria, and an over-bath or level-access shower might be fitted. The temptation is to recommend an adaptation which might be a non-essential and more expensive solution, rather than see the person denied a service.

Alternative funding options

There are certain situations where alternative or part-funding for an adaptation funding should be considered. Some authorities operate top-up budgets to assist with the user contribution in cases of financial hardship, and care management or intermediate care funds should be discussed with care managers when, for instance, a costly residential place or care package is under discussion. A financial contribution might prevent admission altogether or reduce the costs while waiting for an adaptation to be carried out. A transfer of funds from the NHS under Health Acts 1977 and 1999 may be used to speed up hospital discharges, or charitable funding might be explored. Direct payments funding might also be an option to consider where the adaptation would be supported and funded by social care services.

Case study 7.6: care management or intermediate care funds can speed up the process
Mrs C lives with her husband and their supportive family. She has deteriorating mobility and was recently admitted to hospital, received a period of rehabilitation and is now ready to return home when a stairlift can be installed.

A short-term place has been found for her in a nearby residential home (funded from a community care budget) as there is no space for a bed downstairs in her home, but the weekly cost of this will amount to more than the installation of the stairlift. If the normal DFG procedure is followed, it will take several weeks to install.

If alternative funding is used to order the stairlift, she can return home within a very short time and money be saved on her placement.

Users may choose to fund more expensive options themselves. They may have a preference on how their home is to be adapted and wish to bear the difference in cost between that and the occupational therapist's recommendation. Bull (1998b, p. 67), however, cites legal advice against agreement to private arrangements associated with a grant to fund an adaptation that is known to be unsafe.

Occupational therapists need to be aware of budget restrictions and will need to justify to funding authorities and their clinical supervisors their support for a particular adaptation, and this assists in testing clinical reasoning and ensuring that the user has been fully involved in the process. There may be a choice of options, and the relative merits of each should be considered and reasons given why they are/are not suitable in the circumstances.

Occupational therapists should be aware of the Best Value policy that local authorities must adopt and the need for a value-for-money approach to their recommendations. Options may be graded to meet individual needs by as simple and cost-effective a manner as possible, as needs can be met in a variety of ways when deciding what course of action to take.

Occupational therapists, however, often find themselves having to 'fit needs into available resources' and acting as gatekeepers to local authority budgets. FACS guidance (s 23) (DoH, 2002a) sets out very clearly that the use of 'blanket policies' should not be used to determine what services are provided, for instance in restricting provision for bathing to 'medical need only' or to 'basic equipment only' if a strip wash is not possible. The real issue must be whether a person has a need for assistance in maintaining their own personal hygiene and how that need should be met.

The process has so far only dealt with assessing need and preparing an intervention plan. The occupational therapist then assists the disabled user and their carer to reach agreement on how to meet the needs identified in the intervention plan. This involves using an ever-expanding personal knowledge base to find unique solutions and a creative approach to adapting the home environment.

Translating needs into adaptations

Clinical reasoning and problem-solving

Using the same approach as for care planning, the occupational therapist must consider what is meant by 'outcome' (see Chapter 9). Is the outcome the level access shower or stairlift or is it the ability to wash independently or use the stairs?

In determining the desired outcome and how it is to be achieved, the therapist should employ clinical reasoning (see Chapter 3) as well as a user-centred approach to problem-solving. The solution to an environmental problem might appear straightforward but is often complicated by other circumstances; these have to be weighed up and any likely risk reduced to the minimum. This might result in recommending a solution which is more than is required for the assessed need but the only safe option in that situation.

Where agreement on the solution is difficult to reach, the occupational therapist assists the disabled person to reach a solution which satisfies all considerations. There may be technical difficulties, certain risks to safety, options with varying cost implications or the family may have strong preferences. Jensen et al. (1998) observe that considerable time might be needed to consider all options and that often people with evident functional difficulties seem unable to accept the need to plan for future changes. This might delay the process, and using a short-term solution might be more acceptable at the early stages of their disability.

Whatever the considerations, the final adaptation must meet the need and be acceptable to the person concerned. Nocon and Pleace (1997) found that a range of professionals involved with planning adaptations failed to listen to disabled people or agree to their wishes. Research has shown that without this agreement adaptations may therefore not be used at all because they are unacceptable (Heywood, 2001).

User-centred practice: creativity and individualised solutions

Each adaptation is unique, but nevertheless there are certain 'givens' which can lead to clear conclusions: problems posed by stairs may be overcome by a stairlift, an inability to use the bath may indicate a level-access shower, a wheelchair user will need wide doors and level access.

These situations usually meet criteria for funding (they would, for instance, be awarded a mandatory DFG) and the occupational therapist has clear options to discuss.

The following section, however, covers some groups of people needing assistance in adapting their homes where the eligibility and solutions are not so clear. Here the occupational therapist must be convinced of the need and may have to support the individual in establishing their right to funding. It is interesting to note that these examples not only demonstrate how an adaptation can make a difference to the user and carer, including their wider well-being and to the care package, but also allow the occupational therapist to function in a more creative and empowering way.

Children with disabilities

The DFG means test of parents of a disabled child under the age of 16 years (except N. Ireland, which abolished the means test for families with a disabled child in 2003 and the Welsh Assembly in 2005) can result in a high and unaffordable contribution. Research has shown that parents often withdraw from the process, that families experience hardship as a result and children with progressive conditions can experience increasing difficulties in the future (O'Brien, 2003). Occupational therapists working with families in this situation should advise them on alternative funding options and ensure that care managers or other workers are made aware of any concerns resulting from the adaptation not being pursued.

Planning an adaptation requires consideration of both existing and longer-term needs as the child grows up, and the needs of the family must also be taken into account. A study carried out in 2002 reported that lack of space was a frequently reported problem by families, including space for play, for privacy, for equipment use and storage and for therapy (Beresford and Oldman, 2002).

> **Case study 7.7: use of simple changes to reduce strain in a family**
> Mr and Mrs L have two sons aged 8 and 10 years with autistic spectrum disorder and live in a terraced house on an estate close to the main road. Both boys constantly try to leave the house and run away and are unaware of hazards in the home. They require constant supervision at home, and although the parents have regular respite care arrangements, they feel they will soon need help in the home so that they can maintain the safety of both boys.
>
> Adaptations might include a safe play area in the house with a stable (half) door so that the children are visible from outside the room and a double porch or fencing outside. Small alterations, such as self-closing taps in the bathroom, might be considered.

The provision of relatively simple alterations would improve the safety of the boys and leave the parents free to arrange their work commitments and holidays more flexibly. The strain on both parents would be reduced and they may feel less need to call on outside support as a result.

These alterations can be funded by an adaptation budget rather than use of the DFG system or from community care funds, using the Children Act as a basis for provision.

People with deteriorating illness or palliative care needs

A responsive adaptations service in these situations should use speedy and imaginative (short-term) solutions. Prioritising assessments and fast-track agreements with housing or grants officers ensures there are no unnecessary delays. Solutions might have to fit into the existing structure of the house to reduce upheaval and avoid a lengthy building process. Health and social care funding might be used and clear agreements need to be made to avoid delays.

Case study 7.8: short-term solutions provided in a timely way

Mr B is due to return home to live after accepting that he has only a few months left to live. He uses a wheelchair and can transfer at the moment. He lives with his partner and their two young children in their own small terraced house with one living room. The bathroom and separate WC are upstairs. There is no ground-floor space to put a bed and he will need assistance with transfers onto a hospital bed eventually.

Agreement over funding and a flexible approach to this situation could ensure the fitting of a hired stairlift, removal of a partition wall in the bathroom to enlarge it and give access to a wash basin, funded by social care and a hoist gantry for the nurses funded by the Primary Care Trust, who also provide the bed.

The result is that by use of simple solutions the DFG process and lengthy delays have been avoided. Mr B can be nursed at home with dignity and without placing additional stress on the family, thus also avoiding the necessity of a nursing home or hospice bed unless chosen.

People with sensory impairment

Occupational therapists are not expert in this field, but may wish to include sensory impairment needs in an overall adaptation plan. They will want to work closely with the disabled person, who is the expert on their own needs, and to consult specialists working within the authority or from the voluntary sector. Guidance published by the RNIB in Wales (Rees and Lewis, 2004) gives details about falls avoidance and risk reduction, including potential risk in the bathroom, and a home assessment checklist which is comparable to one which might be used for people with physical impairments.

People with learning disabilities

Social role valorisation was developed by O'Brien in the 1980s (O'Brien, 1986), who sought to encourage 'normalisation' for people with learning difficulties and enable them to live, work and spend their leisure time in the community, participate within the community and exercise choice and autonomy. The right to a choice of home and life within it was implicit.

With supportive care packages and funding for changes to the home, families are able to provide care at home for a child or young person with a learning disability, before the decision to move away is made. Within the family context, it is important to take into account the needs of the whole family as well as the individual, and consultation with specialist organisations, advocacy services or workers directly involved can be helpful.

Case study 7.9: an adaptation for the benefit of the whole family
Emma S is a teenager with a learning disability and co-ordination difficulties. She lives with her two teenage siblings and her parents. Mr S works full time and Mrs S works shorter hours to assist Emma in the mornings as she takes a long time, particularly in the bathroom. The family all use one WC, which is in the bathroom, and there is considerable tension in the mornings with her mother suffering from stress as a result. Emma has tried using the bathroom last, but she misses the bus to her school and has to take a taxi funded by social services. Mrs S is now asking for a carer in the mornings and for increased respite arrangements.

The adaptation options to resolve this situation depend upon the layout of the home, what the family believe would ease the situation and whether Emma can be helped to become more independent. It might be possible to separate or enlarge some of the existing facilities for Emma's own use. The opinion of a social worker or teacher would give a perspective on how she might manage.

Once the separate or enlarged facilities are in place, Emma can take the time she needs to get ready, might be able to take the school bus and might become more independent as a result. The stress on the family is reduced, a carer is not required because Emma is more independent, the usual respite arrangements are considered sufficient by the family and the mother might be able to increase her working hours because the process is no longer so long.

People with mental health needs

Dual diagnosis is one possible reason for a housing adaptation, but mental health needs might in themselves require a solution, where the environment is impacting on the person and contributing to the problems. The location of housing for people with mental health needs can be important – whether it is socially isolating, with poor transport or in a hostile neighbourhood; an occupational therapy assessment would take all this into account when assisting with planning a move (Bull, 1998b). Professionals in the mental health field or advocacy services might assist in planning an adaptation with the user and occupational therapist in these situations. Joint risk assessments can determine the level of priority or urgency for the presenting need.

People from minority ethnic groups: addressing cultural diversity

The issues surrounding cultural diversity and the needs of people from different ethnic backgrounds impact on their use of the home. In some cultures the care of an elderly or sick person does not lead to independence as this conflicts with the expectation that family will help (Gibbs and Barnitt, 1999). Some families expect to live in one dwelling, with younger members caring for older ones. This requires more space, which should be recognised (Heywood, 2001). The different ethnic communities observe various rituals and customs of which the therapist must be aware and respect. These might include the need for a prayer area, the need for running water when washing (although this does not necessarily mean a shower), customs associated with toileting and the way food is prepared (Meghani-Wise, 1996). Consultation with local organisations and the use of independent translators or advocacy services are recommended.

> ### Case study 7.10: a solution which allows for independence and respect for religious practice
>
> Mr and Mrs P have three young children and Mr P's elderly mother living in their home. Mr P works, but Mrs P, who would like to work, is unable to do so because her mother-in-law needs help to go upstairs during the day to use the WC. An extra stair rail has been fitted, but it is not sufficient. In order for Mrs P to go out to work and take/collect her children from school, a WC is needed downstairs and meanwhile other family members must visit regularly each day to assist her mother-in-law to climb the stairs.

There is a small space to install a ground-floor WC, but the family currently use it for their prayer area and they are reluctant to accept a commode in the living room because they say it would upset her dignity to use it there.

The installation of a stairlift in this situation means that the elderly woman can now be left alone during the day. She can use the WC when she needs it and no longer needs help to climb the stairs. In addition the family's religious practice has been observed and so has respect and privacy for the older woman.

Adaptations for carers

The needs of the carer must be considered and, although the legislation covers informal (unpaid) carers, the provision of adaptations would be expected to assist formal (paid) carers also. Adaptations can be divided into those changes which increase independence of the individual and thus reduce the effort of the carer or which assist the carer directly, such as the provision of a hoist or extra space allowance in critical areas.

Recommending the adaptation and co-ordinating the work

Once a solution has been identified and agreed with the disabled person, their carer and those agencies involved in providing care, the occupational therapist must state clearly what is required to the authority carrying out the work. When the adaptation is to be funded by a DFG, the occupational therapist must confirm that the work is 'necessary and appropriate' and guidance on this for more complex cases is given by the ODPM (2004c).

The occupational therapist recommendation is accompanied by a customised brief or specification of the needs of the individual, taking into account the user's needs and preferences, functional requirements and psychological and social aspects of care (NIHE, 2003a). Specifications are the translation of needs to achieve a performance outcome and reflect the agreement made with the disabled person during the assessment. They must describe what is required (Bull, 1998b) to avoid confusion or misunderstanding during the process and are the point of reference should the completed work be unsuccessful in any way. Heywood (2001) points out that accurate specifications are fundamental to the success of an adaptation and that this applies to all adaptations irrespective of size. This will have been discussed with the disabled person to avoid disagreements.

Emphasis has been placed on the need for occupational therapists to work closely with care managers and other professionals at the decision-making stage of an adaptation, and it is essential that similar close co-operation continues with other colleagues throughout the process.

Although occupational therapists invariably find themselves acting as co-ordinators or keyworkers during the adaptation process, this is not a core skill and might be seen as a waste of a scarce resource. Those agencies that are partners in adaptation work such as Home Improvement Agencies should be encouraged to take on this role or, alternatively, research has shown that, if given the choice and sufficient information at the early stage of the adaptation process, some disabled people are capable and might prefer to co-ordinate their own adaptation with support (Picking and Pain, 2003).

Conclusion

This chapter has described the role of the occupational therapist in community care services, working with care managers, other professionals and support staff. Occupational therapists from all areas of health and social care must work within tightly controlled legislative frameworks and conflicting funding arrangements to ensure their patients or clients receive a person-centred, needs-led service. This requires a broad skill base and a willingness to look at a situation as widely as possible to find unique solutions.

The occupational therapist looks beyond obvious solutions, identifies and minimises the risks, understands the impact of change upon lives and the implication of one option over another while being ever mindful of cost. A partnership approach is an important part of the process, and occupational therapists can demonstrate that their role is not just about the 'bricks and mortar' of housing but about the assessment of and working with individuals to achieve what they wish for themselves and ensuring other agencies appreciate this.

The user-centred approach means helping people take responsibility for themselves, including taking risks, and maintaining an open mind about the less straightforward situations. Acting not as gatekeeper but as enabler or advocate is crucial to this approach.

Key points

- OTs in local authorities work within the context of care management and are an essential part of community care services.
- Housing is an integral part of community care, and decisions related to adaptations are influenced by this and in turn can impact on the broader package of care.

- All OTs involved with housing adaptations need an understanding of the legal context and range of funding options available to work effectively in this context.
- Partnership working is required to ensure that adaptations can be used to overcome a broad range of needs.
- OTs are encouraged to adopt a creative approach to achieve individualised solutions to meet users' needs.

Acknowledgements

Thanks to Jeremy Cooper, who advised on the legal aspects of this chapter, and Maryanne Cook, Occupational Therapy Team Manager, Hampshire County Council, who also advised on this chapter.

CHAPTER 8

Ergonomics and housing

CARLA BENEDICT, SAMANTHA POOLEY AND
JANI GRISBROOKE

This chapter will explore the usefulness of the ergonomics theory base to occupational therapy practice. The similarities and differences between the focus of OT and ergonomics will be identified along with the resultant need to adapt models and assessments when moving across these disciplinary boundaries. The use of adapted ergonomic models and assessments in OT assessment will be explored, including analysis of information, identification of problems and synthesis of possible solutions. Finally, the impact of anthropometrics (the ergonomic study of sizes and shapes of people in specific populations) and particularly bariatrics (that branch which concentrates on people of more than average size in populations) on OT practice in housing will be explored.

Introduction

The predominant role of a British occupational therapist working for a local authority is to adapt houses for disabled people, which may or may not include assistive technology.

The whole process of adapting property is initiated by the occupational therapist after the referral stage. To use ergonomic terminology they must 'predict, investigate and develop' solutions to adapt a property for a disabled person just as an ergonomist must 'predict, investigate and develop' solutions to adapt working environments (Wilson, 1995).

Both disciplines recognise the need to balance the many influences on this type of work. There are the personal ones of the individuals directly concerned – their abilities, needs and aspirations and then the 'Outside Influences' as described by Wilson (1995), including legal, technical, financial and social issues. Both disciplines are aware that to do this it is essential that a thorough assessment is carried out of the influences, and both disciplines try to achieve the same goal: to provide 'a safe, comfortable, effective and satisfactory' environment for a user (Wilson, 1995). The evaluation of their work is based on whether this goal is achieved.

Other authors, such as Hagedorn (2000) and Corcoran and Gitlin (1997), have written about the use of ergonomic features by an occupational therapist, but few explain when and how to apply them in the field of housing adaptation. This chapter will attempt to do this. Some ergonomic methodology and principles will be explored and appropriate parts utilised and combined with occupational therapy core skills and clinical reasoning to construct a number of frameworks which the occupational therapist can apply in this area of work.

This chapter is divided into four main sections. The first section of the chapter looks at an ergonomic risk assessment for manual handling and adapts it to produce the thorough assessment process needed for housing adaptations. It will be referred to as the 'core assessment' in the rest of this chapter.

The second and third sections will assume the 'core assessment' has been carried out and go on to explore ergonomic theory, which will enable the occupational therapist to extricate the essential parts of the assessment and analyse them to develop solutions.

The fourth section will focus on the relevance of anthropometric data when considering ergonomic factors around housing and the design of built environments and products. Bariatric care is used as an example.

The initial 'core' assessment

An occupational therapist and ergonomist cannot begin to 'predict, investigate and develop' solutions (Wilson, 1995) without adequate information about the situation they need to change. This section looks at what information is required and the ways of obtaining it using an adapted ergonomic approach as a guide.

The approach must be adapted because where there are similarities with the two disciplines, as noted in the introduction to this chapter, there are essential differences as well. The following is a definition of an ergonomic assessment.

> Ergonomics is the subject which looks at how things, jobs, environment etc. are matched to people's sizes, strengths, abilities and other human attributes. It takes the position that situations should be designed primarily for those people involved with them. It is a 'people centred' viewpoint rather than a 'job centred' one. The consequence of good ergonomics in the workplace is more effective, healthier and less stressful work, which is a benefit to everyone. (Corlett and McAtamney, 1992, p. 1)

An occupational therapist can embrace this statement but they would automatically extend its sentiment to the home environment as well as the work environment and would give a different interpretation to some of the terms used, as shown in Table 8.1.

Table 8.1 Comparison of OT and ergonomist approaches

	Ergonomist	Occupational therapist
People-centred	A population of workers	A population of one
Human attributes	Characteristics assigned to a human	Qualities and characteristics of a person
Things	Inanimate objects	Social, psychological, spiritual aspects of life
Workplace	Work environment	Community and workplaces
Work	Employment	Life occupations

Application of an ergonomic risk assessment to occupational therapy in housing

Since the Manual Handling Operations Regulations (MHOR; Great Britain, 1992), the profession has actively used an ergonomic approach to moving and handling risk assessments. The approach is based on the following template:

- load
- other factors
- task
- individual capabilities
- environment

This section will look at how this ergonomic approach to assessment can be adapted for use for the preliminary, core assessment for housing adaptations. The Health and Safety Executive's (HSE, 1992) Guidance on Manual Handling Operations Regulations assessment and Pearce and Cassar (1999) are used to trigger assessment questions.

An ethical warning for OTs using MHOR terminology
One very important difference in using this ergonomic template in occupational therapy housing work is that the MHOR 1992 terminology of *load* becomes *person* to pre-empt any possibility of the assessor viewing the person as an object. Persons possess biomechanical properties but

they cannot be defined solely in those terms or they cease to be persons. OT practice must explore the uniqueness of the individual person in his or her specific life from a basis of respect and with a person-centred approach (COT, 2005).

In the HSE Guidance, 'The Task' is the first factor for assessment. An ergonomist aims to complete a work task efficiently and safely and can alter the load and environment to ensure the task can be done and then pick the individuals with the right human characteristics and train them to do the task. But an occupational therapist is assessing a population of one, a specific individual and so they will consider the 'person' first. With only minor alteration and additions, the checklist that follows is taken from Pearce and Cassar (1999). It provides a very comprehensive aide-memoire for this assessment.

The person

This checklist includes a full range of physical characteristics, impairments, physical parameters and abilities, sensation, cognition, valued roles and occupations and psychological, social and cultural issues:

* age
* gender
* weight, size, shape
* medical condition – is it stable or likely to improve or deteriorate and at what pace
* abnormalities and restricted movements
* vulnerable areas – skin, bone, specific joints, sores, wounds etc.
* weakness, paralysis and impaired muscle tone
* balance, stability, ability to weightbear and for how long and with what support
* ability to step and walk and with what support
* wheelchair user – full-time/part-time, what type and size
* co-ordination
* hypersensitive areas or loss of sensation or awareness of body parts
* frequency or history of dizzy spells or falling
* continence
* attachments, splints, braces, catheters, stoma bags, drips, drains etc.
* equipment used
* ability to understand, follow instructions, feedback and communicate
* sight, hearing and speech
* memory and confusion
* cultural considerations, modesty, fear

- essential and leisure occupations
- roles and relationships such as worker or mother
- challenging behaviour

Other factors

Every experienced occupational therapist working in the field of housing adaptations knows that it can appear, at first glance, quite obvious how to adapt a property to achieve a good physical result. This occupational therapist also knows that 'first glance' proposals to adapt a property for a disabled person may well be rejected by that person and those close to them because *other factors* have not been considered.

In this adapted core assessment *other factors* has an entirely different meaning to the *other factors* in an ergonomic risk assessment. The importance of this category to occupational therapists is alongside that of the *person* category. Here the occupational therapy and ergonomic disciplinary focus again diverge with occupational therapy taking a specifically person-centred approach and valuing all the unique characteristics of this person and his or her situation which makes them different to any other. As Professor Keith Bright, Department of Construction Management and Engineering Research Group for Inclusive Environments, University of Reading, said, 'OTs have skills which are not found in the design industry' (COTSSIH, 2003).

Other factors will include:

- the person's 'hierarchy of importance of occupations' both essential and leisure or, put another way, their needs and aspirations;
- personal preferences;
- impact of spatial design on family routines and family dynamics (NB. family here stands for network of significant people rather than genetic or marital kinship);
- how the person views a deteriorating medical condition or an acquired impairment;
- meanings of home and spatial design for the person and significant others.

Case study 8.1

We had the best possible level-access shower installed to meet my bathing requirements. On the surface of it this suited my physical needs perfectly, but it was a disaster in every other way. As someone who had been in institutions from the age of 18 months to 19 years, I had suffered all manner of violence and abuse, mostly in the bathroom and a lot of it in showers.

'Best adaptation can only happen if a person's specialist needs emerge from a sensitive and holistic assessment of who they are and what kind of life they wish to lead.' (Winfield, 2003, p. 376)

The task

The assessment of tasks requires the occupational therapist to analyse a whole range of tasks of daily living – personal, domestic, leisure and work. A task analysis involves breaking down a task into component parts:

- The sequence – the stages of the task and in what order these are tackled.
- The method – describes how each part of the task is done.
- The content – asks why a task is being carried out and what is being produced and what is required to achieve it. (Hagedorn, 2000)

The questions posed in the HSE Guidance (1992), along with some additional questions relating to cognitive ability, indicate the information needed for analysis of tasks to be completed without the assistance of another.

The task – does it involve the following?

- holding loads away from the trunk
- twisting
- stooping
- reaching upwards
- large vertical movements
- long carrying distances
- strenuous pushing and pulling
- unpredictable movement of loads
- repetition handling
- insufficient rest or recovery
- a workrate imposed by a process
- cognitive ability – reasoning skills, memory, concentration, persistence, previous knowledge

The list below is taken from Pearce and Cassar (1999) and can be used when analysing a task completed with the assistance of another.

The task – what has to be done and what factors are involved?

- Is the task necessary?
- How much is the person contributing?
- Is the task repetitive?
- What postures are being adopted?
- Is there a need to stoop, reach, twist or hold a load away from the body? Or is there a need to maintain an awkward posture?
- Is this one single task or is this one of many tasks?
- How long does the task take?

- How many people are required to assist?
- What equipment is used?
- Is the task necessary?

Task analysis can be carried out using different methods, but whatever method is used, the analysis has its limitations because it does not take into account less tangible aspects such as a person's mood or variation in ability during the day and from day to day.

Individual capability

If the task analysis reveals the need for someone to assist the person to complete a task, then the occupational therapist will need to assess what individual capabilities are required to do this. The HSE Guidance's (1992) questions are the most useful here:

- Does the task require unusual capability – strength or height, for instance?
- Is it a hazard to those with a health problem?
- Does it call for special information/training?

This assessment may contribute to how the accommodation is adapted and whether part of the adaptation is the introduction of specialist equipment, such as ceiling track hoist or glide-about commode.

Environment

Having assessed the *person* and analysed the *tasks* that person needs and wishes to carry out, the occupational therapist must assess the *environment* where the tasks will be performed.

This is another part of the assessment which is largely specific to the occupational therapist; a few key questions can be used from the HSE Guidance (1992), but in order to plan the changes required the occupational therapist must:

- know who owns the accommodation;
- have a ground plan of the accommodation;
- have detailed scale drawings of key areas;
- have details of floor levels, ventilation, heating and lighting.

Using each heading – *person, other factors, tasks, individual capabilities* and *environment*, the information required for this core assessment is gathered.

There is more than one way of collecting the information, including discussion with all concerned, the use of diaries or video and audio recordings, photographic recording and questionnaires (Wilson, 1995). In every instance, they must include the observation of physical abilities, scale drawings and the client's hierarchy of importance of occupations, both leisure and essential.

Housing adaptations can be large and complex projects, involving people other than the client. Mistakes may be irretrievable and so thorough assessment is essential – 'The devil is in the detail.'

The ergonomic risk assessment template is a useful one to use when assessing for housing adaptations because it helps to ensure detailed information is gathered and then organised into compartments which can be analysed as part of the process to produce successful recommendations for housing adaptations. The next two sections consider the analysis of the information gained from this assessment.

Applying an adapted ergonomic model to analyse assessment findings

The model in Figure 8.1 has been devised, by the author, to provide the occupational therapist with a framework to analyse the information obtained from the core assessment as described in the previous section and from this analysis develop solutions so that a housing adaptation is successful. It uses the terminology and sequence of an ergonomic model (Buckle and Randle, 1989).

To illustrate the use of this adapted ergonomic model, a complex case is considered. It is complicated because the *person* had both cognitive

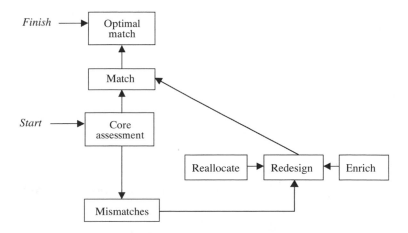

Figure 8.1 Ergonomic model. Source: adapted from Buckle and Randle (1989).

and physical problems due to a traumatic incident, and one of the major consequences was a change in her personal relationships.

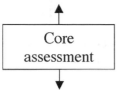

The model started with the 'Core Assessment', with all the information gathered under the previously described headings of *person*, *other factors*, *the task*, *individual capabilities* and *environment*.

The person (here known as Mary)

Mary was a 42-year-old woman who experienced a traumatic brain injury as a result of a road traffic accident.

- 5ft 7in tall, of slim build, weighing 10.5 stone.
- Affected both cognitively and physically.
- At the time of referral she was an in-patient at a rehabilitation centre.

Cognitive involvement

- Short attention span.
- Poor short-term memory.
- Exhibited obsessive behaviour – she had to be actively involved with the laundering and care of her clothes.
- She felt disorientated in large rooms, preferring a square-shaped room.
- She felt more comfortable and able if items she needed to complete a task were within her vision.

Upper- and lower-limb involvement

- She had an upper-limb weakness and loss of sensation on the left side. She had some gross movements in the left hand but no strength or dexterity. She was right-handed.
- She could stand with assistance but unable to turn her feet once standing or walk independently.
- Used a battery-operated wheelchair inside and outside.

Occupation

- Garden designer – she had worked from home.

Social situation

- She had lived with her long-term partner (here known as Paul) in a house they owned.
- No children.
- She had enjoyed playing tennis and the theatre.

Other factors

- Paul felt the relationship had been failing since before the accident and he did not want to be involved in any personal care tasks for Mary and so he took the decision to change his role from partner to advocate. He moved out of the home they had shared.
- Mary was, initially, unaware of her changed status and that her partner had moved out of their shared home. She seemed very dependent on his support and frequent visits to the rehabilitation centre.
- The occupational therapist at the rehabilitation centre worked with Mary to compile a 'hierarchy of importance of occupation'. This ran as follows:
  - independence in personal care tasks;
  - ability to prepare meals, snacks and drinks;
  - she was insistent that she was involved with laundering and care of clothes;
  - return to her job as a garden designer.
- She was unable to accept that her physical limitations might prevent her from achieving her desires.

The task

Task analysis was required of the tasks she most wanted to be able to do and to establish what would be required to enable her to do them. Task analysis was carried out by observation, reports from the occupational therapist in the rehabilitation centre and questionnaires completed by the rehabilitation centre's occupational therapist and Paul.

Task analysis is key to developing a *redesign*.

Individual capabilities

Task analysis would reveal what was required of others to assist Mary.

Environment

- Power points were just above floor level and the light switches and window heights were set at a height for a standing person.
- There was a short drive at the front and large gardens to the side and back of the house.
- Mary worked from a garden house at the bottom of the garden.

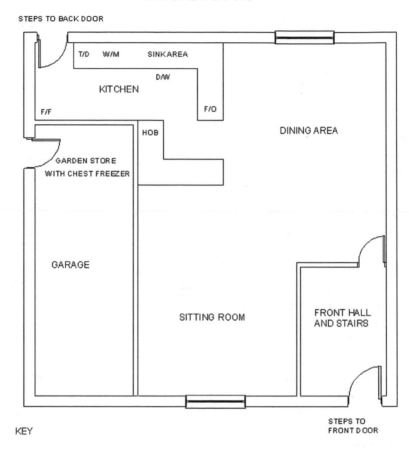

GROUND FLOOR

Figure 8.2 Drawing of Mary's house before adaptation (not to scale).

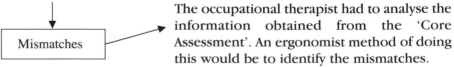

Mismatches

The occupational therapist had to analyse the information obtained from the 'Core Assessment'. An ergonomist method of doing this would be to identify the mismatches. There are two types of mismatches:

• The personal ones – the *person's* abilities may not 'match' what abilities are required to complete the *tasks* they need or desire to achieve in the *environment* in which they live.

- The *person's* aspirations may not match *outside influences*: they may not be legally compliant, financially viable, societally acceptable or technically sound (Wilson, 1995).

Mary's mismatches

On referring to the scale drawing of her home, the environmental mismatches were apparent. She was unable to:

- access her home from the outside;
- reach the upper floor, bedroom and bathroom;
- use existing bathroom facilities;
- independently access all the rooms in her home;
- access and carry out tasks in the kitchen;
- access the garden house at one end of her garden;
- access the garden and carry out any garden tasks.

Her cognitive involvement revealed a number of mismatches between her desires and her physical and cognitive abilities.

- To be involved in every aspect of caring for her clothes.
- To be independent in personal care and meal preparation tasks.
- To return to her job as a garden designer.
- Disorientation in large rooms, preferring square-shaped ones, and yet space would be needed for wheelchair use.

Mary was unaware of the social change that had occurred – Paul's change of role from partner to advocate. This meant there was a mismatch between Mary's expectations of the future, which still involved having a partner, and the reality. The revelation of this would be very painful for Mary; her whole 'life plan' had been jeopardised. Careful management of this change by the occupational therapist, working with others, would be needed to salvage some of it; some of 'the salvage' could be in the housing adaptation.

Because Paul was such a strong influence in the case, we must highlight his mismatches as well.

Paul's mismatches

The change of role from partner to advocate was a very difficult one for Paul. This influenced his contribution towards the planning of the adaptation and caused a mismatch. He appeared to compensate for his decision by being very confrontational and demanding to all involved with the process of adapting the property. He wanted to retain the house as it was downstairs and extend upstairs to give Mary a shower room and facilities for any carers involved.

Outside influences' mismatches

These refer to the legal, financial, societal and technical influences involved with an adaptation. In this particular case an example of a legal and financial influence was 'Part 1 of the Housing Grants, Construction and Regeneration Act 1996' because the occupational therapist would refer to the environmental health department of the local council for a Disabled Facilities Grant. The Act specifies the types of work that can be undertaken to qualify for a Disabled Facilities Grant and requires them to be 'necessary' and 'appropriate'; this caused a mismatch with regard to Paul's aspirations.

The Act also requires the work to be 'reasonable' and 'practicable'; this refers to the technical requirements of a proposal; sometimes these are very complex and the end result does not justify 'the means'. In this example, Paul's desire to retain the house as it was downstairs and to extend the upstairs was technically possible but complicated and costly.

A moment to consider the impact of using this model so far
The model provided the occupational therapist with a 'pathway' through what was a jungle of hard facts, needs and aspirations. They identified not only the physical and environmental mismatches but also the less tangible ones, It provided the process of analysis and prioritisation of the information.

This adaptation required other professionals to be involved such as surveyors and grant officers. These professionals considered the physical and environmental mismatches but did not fully appreciate the less tangible ones, which had as much significance. It was the role of the occupational therapist to present these *other factors* where necessary and indicate their level of importance to ensure they were part of the equation when the adaptation of the property was planned.

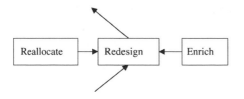

Mary's needs, aspirations and abilities were considered along with the identified 'mismatches' and the solutions developed were more than a redesign of her home.

Enrich

Specialist equipment would be part of the *enrich*, to assist Mary to achieve her aspirations. However, rehabilitation revealed that even with equipment and adaptation to the property Mary would be unable to complete a number of essential tasks, and so another part of the *enrich* was that a live-in carer/enabler would be employed. This needed to be taken into account in the *redesign*. The occupational therapist worked with the rehabilitation team to assess the 'individual capabilities' the carer/enabler would require to assist Mary.

Reallocation

Reallocation not only referred to tasks being reallocated from Paul and Mary but tasks being reallocated a different status, for instance gardening would initially be a hobby as opposed to a work task and clothes management would be raised from a low-priority task to a high one.

Redesign

The occupational therapist established that the following should be included in any adaptation carried out:

- Wheelchair access to the dwelling would be through the rear of the property so Mary would also gain access to the garden.
- Doorways would be wheelchair accessible.
- The kitchen would be adapted for wheelchair manoeuvrability and seated work. Mary would need access to most areas in the kitchen and be able to achieve optimum positioning with regard to her medical condition. There needed to be sufficient room for the carer/enabler to be seated by Mary to assist her and an area where the carer/enabler could stand to work. Special emphasis would be placed on the positioning of clothes washing and drying facilities.
- A level-access shower room would be provided with a wheelchair-accessible basin and automatic wash/dry type toilet to promote as much independence as possible for Mary in the bathroom. An attendant push shower chair would be used in the shower area and over the toilet so once positioned Mary would be independent.
- A ceiling tracked hoist would be required in the bedroom for transfers to bed, wheelchair and shower chair. (The *individual capabilities* assessment revealed this was required.)
- A separate bedroom and bathroom would be required for a live-in carer/enabler.
- Facilities provided so Mary could continue with garden design as a hobby initially but as work, perhaps, in the future.

All options needed to include the special requirements of Mary as identified in *other factors* such as the shapes and layouts of rooms, for example, as many working areas as possible were square-shaped.

Options considered

Part of the *redesign* was to consider all the options available and consider them in detail.

Option 1: Wheelchair access to the upper floor via a through floor lift

This was discounted because:

- The ceilings upstairs were sloped, which would have made installation of a ceiling tracked hoist very difficult.
- There were only two bedrooms and one bathroom. It was essential that separate facilities away from Mary were provided for the live-in carer/enabler. This would provide privacy for both and encourage the carer/enabler to stay longer in Mary's employment.

Option 2: Paul's option

This was to extend the house over the garage to provide a bedroom and shower room upstairs, accessed via a through floor lift. This would have required extensive work to the roof and an upper-floor extension as well as the downstairs adaptations to the kitchen and access points and so this was rejected on the grounds of being more than was 'necessary and appropriate' and not 'reasonable and practicable' (Part 1 of the Housing Grant, Construction and Regeneration Act 1996).

Option 3: Conversion of the garage and utility room into a downstairs bedroom and level-floor shower room

This option was the most viable because it provided:

- a one-level living area with appropriate facilities so Mary could be as independent as possible with activities and movement;
- a separate space for a live-in carer/enabler to have their own bedroom and bathroom upstairs;
- a spare bedroom for family and friends to stay overnight. This was vital for Mary with the change of her status to a single person.

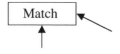

The model then moved to *match* and the occupational therapist was able to check that all the changes proposed would convert as many of the *mismatches* to *matches* as was practicable. It also allowed the revaluation of any unresolved mismatches.

Paul's mismatch of his attitude towards the adaptation and his own plan was overcome by ensuring he was an essential part of the design team. The occupational therapist provided him with scale drawings of rooms along with furniture and equipment templates and always explained and finalised her recommendations along with his before forwarding them to the other professionals. Because he was well informed and felt part of the team developing the redesign, he showed an ability to compromise. He understood the reasons why not all the mismatches had

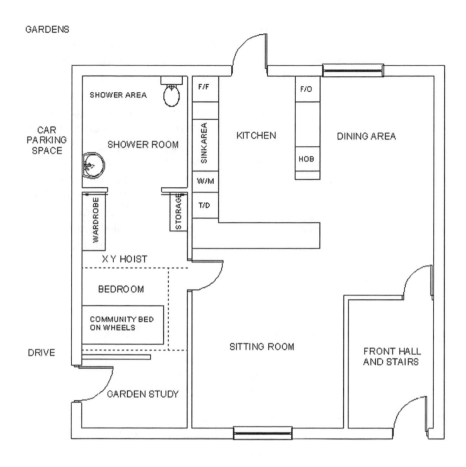

GARDENS

CAR PARKING SPACE

DRIVE

SHOWER AREA

SHOWER ROOM

WARDROBE

X Y HOIST

BEDROOM

COMMUNITY BED ON WHEELS

GARDEN STUDY

F/F

SINK AREA

W/M

T/D

STORAGE

KITCHEN

HOB

F/O

DINING AREA

SITTING ROOM

FRONT HALL AND STAIRS

KEY

F/F - FRIDGE/FREEZER
T/D - TUMBLE DRIER
W/M - WASHING MACHINE
D/W - DISHWASHER
F/O - FITTED OVEN

Figure 8.3 Drawing of Mary's house after adaptation (not to scale).

been converted to matches and as a result decided that he would pay for some enhanced adaptations to the property such as:

- the wall at the end of the bedroom to provide a separate study;
- full glazed door from the study to the garden; this would be the main access to the study area;
- wheelchair-accessible pathways throughout the garden;
- extra raised flower and vegetable beds.

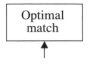

The model allowed the occupational therapist to state clearly what the proposed adaptation would achieve and where there were still mismatches that could not be overcome. In this case Paul contributed to converting some of these outstanding mismatches to matches and with this contribution an *optimal match* was achieved. This *optimal match* could be measured by the end result of a safe, effective, comfortable and satisfactory environment for Mary.

The model highlights the stages necessary to achieve a successful major adaptation. It illustrates that it is essential for the occupational therapist to be aware of how the people involved are reacting to the need to change and what is perceived as a mismatch by the client, those involved with them and the professionals. It enables the occupational therapist to prioritise and focus on the most essential requirements and consider how to compromise and manage the others so that a property can be redesigned to an optimal match.

Applying ergonomic principles of design or redesign

A traditional view of ergonomics is that it is concerned with interactions between people and the things they use and the environments in which they use them. (Wilson, 1995, p. 8)

In this section another ergonomic principle (Figure 8.4) will be adapted by the author to provide the occupational therapist with a framework in which to analyse housing adaptation options (Figure 8.5). It could be used as part of the *mismatch* and *redesign* stages of the model used in the second section, for complex cases, or stands alone for less complicated cases.

This approach will be adapted here to assist an occupational therapist in investigating the best option to overcome the problem of stair climbing.

The core assessment in the first section will have been applied and the option of a second banister or moving to live on the ground floor assessed as inappropriate. The options of the installation of a stairlift or a through floor lift need to be investigated. The installation of the stairlift will be used to illustrate the use of this adapted model. The use of these ergonomic principles will allow the occupational therapist to organise the information gained from the application of the core assessment from the first section in such a way that they will be able to see if the proposed environmental changes will successfully interact with the individual's needs, attributes and aspirations.

The second figure has been adapted to reflect the fact that an individual in their home environment and a specific piece of equipment are being analysed rather than the work environment.

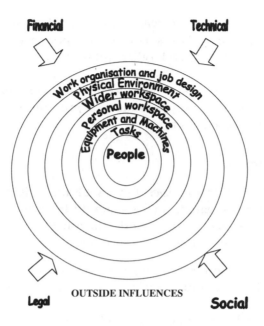

Figure 8.4 Some of the key interactions relevant to work design. Source: Wilson (1995). Printed with permission from Professor John R Wilson and Taylor & Francis Publishers.

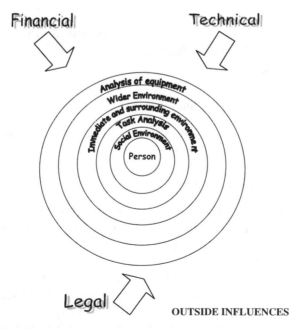

Figure 8.5 Some of the key interactions relevant to housing adaptation. Model adapted from Wilson (1995).

Each layer of this 'onion skin' will be investigated starting at the centre and working to the outside. All layers have equal importance, and the aim is that all interact successfully with each other and with the 'Outside influences'.

The person – this information would have been gained from the core assessment as presented in the first section of this chapter.

Social environment

In this layer factors from *other factors* of the original assessment are investigated. Analysis should be made of the impact the installation of a stairlift may have on the person and those they live with, for example:

- confirming the deterioration of a person's condition;
- confirming the deterioration of a person's condition to those close to them;
- a loss of control to the person and others;
- causing conflict between members of the household;
- concern re safety of other members of the household using the stairs.

But it should:

- allow a disabled person to sleep upstairs where they feel safe;
- allow access to the whole house;
- retain existing room layout.

Task analysis

In this example the occupational therapist would analyse the task of using a stairlift.

In order to use a stairlift independently the person must be able to:

- reach the bottom or the top of the stairs from other parts of the house;
- deposit and retrieve walking aids – if these are to be used, they will be required at the top and bottom of the stairs;
- summon the lift;
- position the seat, footplate and armrests appropriately for transfer on; the seat and footplate may move together or independently; if the latter, the person must be able to access the footplate;
- transfer onto and off the stairlift at both top and bottom of staircase; the seat height is often higher at the base of the stairs than at the top

of the stairs (part of the assessment must be to mimic these heights and try them out with the person); if the footplate and seat are synchronised, then the person is unable to position themselves so, before they sit down, they can 'feel the seat with the back of their legs', the method traditionally used in rehabilitation to encourage the person to obtain a good seated position by sitting back in the seat; the person will, therefore, need to have the ability to position themselves right back on the seat when they are seated and then maintain the position;

- sit with their feet on the footplate and maintain the position;
- manage the hand controls, which require a constant pressure, while the lift travels up and down the stairs;
- manage a manual or powered swivel seat, if one is used, at the top of the stairs;
- manage an automatic fold-down track, if used.

If the person is unable to do any of these tasks, then consideration must be given to whether it is appropriate for another person to assist. If this is the case, the *individual capability* part of the core assessment should be applied to the person assisting.

Special areas of consideration must be:

- If the person needs assistance to transfer onto the stairlift at the base of the stairs, then the carer will be behind the person at the top of the stairs, and will need to get past them in order to assist them to transfer off – this may be impossible.
- If a swivel seat is used at the top of the stairs, then consideration must be given to how the swivel seat will be operated and whether an automatic swivel seat is required.
- The person will be dependent on another person to move about the house and possibly access toilet facilities.
- There is often little room at the top of the stairs for an assistant to position themselves appropriately.

The immediate environment

For the next two layers the information gained from the assessment of environment section needs to be investigated.

The stairs and the immediate space around the staircase consideration should be given to:

- whether the staircase is curved, spiral or with a half landing or complete turn;
- is there sufficient space in the landing areas at the top and bottom of the stairs?
- are any doors positioned at the base of the stairs?
- how wide is the staircase?
- is there sufficient headroom?

The wider environment

By installing a stairlift the problem of climbing the stairs will be overcome, but are there other problems such as access to the home and the outside environment or with bathing and toileting facilities?

Analysis of the equipment

The final layer is an analysis of the equipment itself.

Stairlifts

Assessments are required as to the best type of stairlift and all the accessories. Assistive technology databases such as the Hamilton Index from the Disabled Living Foundation (380–384 Harrow Road, London W9 2HU) may be consulted to obtain more detailed information.

* There are different types – seated, standing platform, perching stool seat and platform.
* There are different tracks – spiral, curved, fill in platform, hinged manual or automatic.
* There are different controls – push button, toggle, joystick and wander lead.
* There are different seats – swivel to different degrees, front-facing, side-facing, foldaway armrests and harnesses.

There are exceptions to every rule but generally if a person cannot use a stairlift independently then an alternative solution should be considered. If there is no alternative and someone must assist, then very careful assessment of the *individual capabilities* of that person must be carried out.

If a person is assessed as not being able to manage the stairs, then a stairlift should cover the whole staircase; it is better not to be tempted to install a stairlift to cover the main body of the staircase leaving some steps out; in the long run this is often foolhardy.

Outside influences

Outside the 'onion' are the financial, technical and legal influences. These will be considered here only in relation to this example.

In Britain, most disabled people requiring major adaptation to their homes will apply for a Disabled Facilities Grant from their local council. This grant is, at the time of writing, mandatory for specific access purposes and of an amount up to but not exceeding £25,000 if the person meets the criteria of eligibility for the grant. The process of application includes a statutory test of the person's financial means to determine if none, part or all of the grant will be funded from public monies. On occasion the means test results in the applicant having to make a contribution towards the costs, which can be difficult or quite impracticable for that applicant to afford (Mandelstam, 1997).

In the example used here it would be unwise to try to compensate for a financial shortfall by installing a stairlift which did not fulfil the needs highlighted in the assessment such as:

* installing a stairlift instead of level-floor accommodation or a through floor lift.
* installing a stairlift on the straight run of the stairs instead of covering the whole staircase.

The range of funding solutions would need to be discussed with a manager.

* The grant officer may consider a discretionary increase to the grant to cover the costs over and above the £25,000 maximum for the mandatory grant.
* Social services may assist by undertaking some of the work needed themselves or giving a top-up grant.
* Charities will sometimes contribute if the statutory authorities have fulfilled all their mandatory obligations.
* Second-hand lifts are available.
* Lifts can be hired.

After the occupational therapist has carried out a full assessment of need and requirements, technical advice may be needed, such as: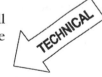

* the width and angles of the staircase;
* the headroom;
* weight limits on track and folding track if appropriate.

 With regard to the example used here, the following British legislation will have been used:

* Part 1 of the Housing Grants, Construction and Regeneration Act 1996, for the Disabled Facilities Grant.

The assessment carried out by the occupational therapist will come under:

- National Assistance Act 1948 – requiring disabled registration;
- Section 2 of the Chronically Sick and Disabled Persons Act 1970;
- NHS and Community Care Act 1990;
- Manual Handling Operations Regulations 1992;
- The Human Rights Act 1998;
- Carers (Recognition and Services) Act 1995.

The model in Figure 8.5 could be used to investigate and predict the successful interaction of features of other adaptations:

- the installation of a ceiling tracked hoist versus a mobile one;
- the installation of a level-floor shower versus retaining the bath with a suitable bathaid or ceiling tracked hoist;
- the installation of extensive ramping versus an outdoor lift.

The occupational therapist can change the titles and order of the interactions in the layers to make them appropriate to the options they are considering; in fact, this is part of the analysis process.

This ergonomic design principle for successful interaction between human elements and environmental elements allows the occupational therapist to analyse thoroughly the information they have gained from an assessment and to investigate the options available. This should ensure a successful outcome of comfort, safety, effectiveness and satisfaction for the disabled person and those involved with them.

Anthropometrics and bariatrics

Models are not the only important aspect of ergonomics. Critical to design is an appreciation of the types of people who will be using the environment or item designed.

Anthropometric data

Anthropometrics is one of the many specialist areas employed by ergonomists to understand the size, shape and proportions of the human body, and the functional inter-relationships within everyday activity, thus providing a baseline from which to design work systems or environments. In order to define a user population and therefore find a design appropriate for reasonably fitting a majority, designers of working systems need to have some idea of the population they are trying to design for.

Since the 1950s, research has led to a broadly accepted anthropometric database. Much of this information has been collated by the Office of Population Censuses and Surveys (OPCS), but perhaps the most quoted in terms of a standard table is the work produced by Stephen Pheasant (1986) concerning statistical description of human variability, and further estimated figures for the bodily dimensions of the adult population of the UK (Pheasant, 1996). The details and ongoing analysis around this work provides standard sources for reference to such anthropometric data, and standards from which further research can be based.

With such information available, manufacturers create products on the basis that they are suitable for most users and choose standard sizes to make goods suitable for mass production and mass consumption. Moving and handling equipment is no exception, and, while all manufacturers will supply bespoke designs for individuals, for example special slings, the standard sizes of small, medium or large are always a more cost-effective option. This could lead to a degree of compromise should the difference between standard size and ideal size for the person be considered as negligible. However, the long-term outcome for the user may not be satisfactory.

While the focus for such statistical analysis is to suit the majority, the minority who are not suited will also be identified. Once this information is obtained, possible solutions for this minority can be investigated, and the impact of problems caused by focusing design on suiting the statistical majority may be minimised for the minority group. For health professionals involved with ergonomic assessment and design, it is this minority population that is of interest since it is within this category that many of our service users fall. People with disabilities, exceptionally small or large people (within defined groups, for example, exceptionally large child or especially small adult), or people who require unusual aids or equipment to achieve or maintain independence are what would be considered 'limiting users' (Pheasant, 1991). If a design is suitable for the majority, it is unlikely that these users will find working systems suitable for their needs.

British Standards (BS) for design of accessible environments are used by architects when planning a new-build or refurbishing an existing facility. However, these are also based on best estimates or suggested plans, and are often too ambiguous to be able to relate details to individual cases, or can even be misleading. For example, BS 8300:2001 12.4.4 suggests that urinals accessible to wheelchair users and ambulant disabled people should provide vertical and horizontal grab rails for the users; this does not consider the possibility that neither may be suitable. In some instances very specific details are given to the precise fixing position, that is lateral position of vertical grab rails should be set 470 mm from the centre line of the toilet, which could prove highly impractical for some. There is no single design that will suit all, but by acknowledging individual difference it can be possible to design appropriately. Occupational therapists use BS as a guide, but, as they work with individual service users, the BS can only inform assessment, not direct it. Another layer of assessment with the particular service user needs to consider a range of specifics such as the distances involved, where the rail would be and/or any limitation in movement.

While it may seem that the application of anthropometrics for those individuals with very specific needs is limited, it is a highly effective way of demonstrating the need for an increased awareness in the initial design parameters, and ensuring the correct user population are defined in the first place. In designing an accessible bathroom, for instance, assumptions will be made about the ability of the user population, and the details around what Pheasant terms 'the four cardinal constraints of anthropometrics' (Pheasant, 1996, p. 22) could provide a clear focus for planning while reducing the potential for unsuitability with the user population.

- *Clearance* – headroom, legroom, access through and around obstacles. Planning an accessible bathroom for full-time wheelchair users will require consideration of basin heights enabling easy access. Handles, fittings and fixtures need to provide adequate apertures for use.
- *Reach* – include location of controls, fixtures, storage areas and/or situational differences, i.e. differing reach capacity if in electric or manual wheelchair.
- *Posture* – locations of controls and displays at the heights of working surfaces: a shower fitting, for example, will determine the postural requirements and therefore constraints imposed. The relationship between bodily dimensions and those of the environment will determine the resultant posture.
- *Strength* – careful consideration needs to be given to what constitutes excessive demands, and there may be difficulty identifying the limiting user. The variations of force application could require strength constraints for both extremes of user, particularly in potentially high-risk environments such as wet rooms.

Perhaps the most difficult of situations arises when there are more complex needs relating to individual circumstances beyond familiar or detailed standards. Designing or adapting an environment for a user population with obesity issues could prove to involve knowledge far beyond usual therapeutic parameters. Knowledge about the load-bearing capacity and structural implications involved in planning such adaptations is the speciality of structural surveyors or engineers, but, if they are not fully aware of the potential physical and practical implications, vital information could be missed. For example, if a person weighing 25 stones requires 24-hour bed care with two carers assisting, the bed must be able to take the weight of all three and the floor must bear the loads involved in a heavy-duty bed provision as well as the potential maximum use. Heavy-duty hoisting equipment may also be required but again it is imperative that the company supplying the equipment are given exact details and specifications to enable the consideration of reinforcement of joists and fixtures at the design stage rather than as a later addition.

To conclude, anthropometrics is intrinsically linked with the ergonomics of posture, movement and environmental analysis. It aims to provide at the very least a guide to the most efficient and effective execution of a functional task, and in doing so provide standards for the guidance of those planning the systems to enable the optimal performance of that task.

Ergonomics and bariatric care

The word 'bariatric' comes from the Greek word *baros* (weight) plus *iatric* (medical treatment), and the term 'bariatric care' is now commonly used by health professionals when planning intervention for heavier people. Bariatrics is a field of medicine that offers treatment for the person who is overweight with a comprehensive programme including diet and nutrition, exercise, behaviour modification, lifestyle changes and, when indicated, the prescription of appropriate medications. Bariatrics also includes research into obesity, its causes, prevention and treatment. Much of this has been led by the USA where adult obesity is now a national problem necessitating a National Task Force on Prevention and Treatment of Obesity (NIDDK, 2004).

The British population is now beginning to mirror this cultural phenomenon, as a House of Commons Health Committee (2004) report illustrates. This report looks at influencing factors and strategies for prevention, highlighting issues around an increasing population of obese people, and the resulting increase in disability.

The impact on social care provision is now becoming apparent as recent tabloid headlines of '40 st man trapped' (*Sun*, July 2004), and '34 st woman stuck on sofa' (*Sun*, August 2004) illustrate. Such articles are obviously reporting dramatic cases where a situation has hit crisis point and any occupational therapy intervention at this point can only be to assist in crisis management such as advocating for the individual concerned, assisting emergency services with transporting a bariatric patient using ergonomic principles and co-ordinating any action plan. Contributing to prevention of such tragic circumstances is where an occupational therapist involved in housing adaptations and specialist equipment provision can play an essential role.

Occupational therapists are often restricted in the solutions available through adaptation, partly as a result of past anthropometric data collection, and the resultant influence this has on current lifestyles. This can be particularly evident when considering the impact on an individual in need of bariatric equipment, that is someone needing special equipment or adaptations as a result of their obesity. The environment in which they live was designed and built with the average person's size, shape and living space requirements in mind.

To appreciate fully the implications of caring for an obese person, that is someone weighing in excess of 25 st (159 kg) (Rush, 2004), a brief case study is given highlighting the impact on ergonomic considerations and housing issues.

Case study 8.2

Background

Mr N is a 44-year-old man who has Chronic Obstructive Airways Disease (COAD); he weighs 29 st and is approximately 6 ft. He lives with his mother, who provides all of his care. Mr N spends most of his time in a riser recliner chair, which is in the main living area, and he is unable to access other rooms due to obstacles and narrow doorways. Mr N is no longer able to negotiate his way to his room, get into his bed or use the bathroom.

Issues/needs

The riser recliner chair Mr N has is not working and is fixed in a semi-recline position; it no longer rises and therefore application of biomechanical principles is practically impossible.

As well as there being a great deal of furniture to negotiate in a room 13 ft × 15 ft, all of the doorways are standard width and no longer accessible, including the bedroom and bathroom. As this difficulty has increased, the desire to move has decreased, and Mr N agrees that it has led to an even more sedentary lifestyle. This in turn has led to further weight gain and long episodes of depression.

Mr N has a bed in another room but this is also beyond repair, is too low and narrow and hasn't been used for over a year. Fortunately, Mr N lives in a ground-floor flat but the floors will have to be checked as the weights and limits involved may exceed safe working loads, as is the case with any equipment that is provided.

Action/solutions

1. Provision of heavy-duty riser recliner chair.
2. Adapting property to have wider doorways to improve accessibility.
3. Provision of a heavy-duty profiling bed to enable independent change of position and enable independent transfers.

4. To make the bathroom and toilet accessible with a heavy-duty commode/shower chair.
5. Application of anthropometric analysis to appropriate systems and equipment. This may enable increased activity, the opportunity for greater energy expenditure, increased manoeuvrability and potential psychosocial benefit as a result of regaining some control within the physical environment at home.

Conclusion

This chapter has been concerned with the importance of the occupational therapist in the process of housing adaptation for disabled people. The four sections have combined ergonomic principles and methodology with occupational therapy core skills and clinical reasoning to develop a number of frameworks and theories that can be used by occupational therapists in this area of work.

Key points

- Occupational therapy can use ergonomic methodology, providing it is a version adapted to support the occupational therapy perspective.
- Occupational therapy is about a holistic approach to housing adaptation – what is technically sound, legally compliant and financially viable must be considered with the needs, abilities and aspirations of the individual person.
- Ergonomics contains a range of disciplinary subsections. Given current social demographics showing an increase in the incidence of obesity, bariatrics is an area of ergonomics which will impact significantly on occupational therapy practice.

Acknowledgements:

Thanks to Nicola Vant for graphics and Amanda White for help with critique.

Professor John R Wilson and Taylor & Francis, publishers, for permission to use Wilson (1995) model cited in chapter.

Professor Peter Buckle and the University of Surrey for permission to use Buckle and Randle (1989) model cited in chapter.

CHAPTER 9

Evaluation for service users and service performance

SUE PENGELLY AND ANDREW WINFIELD

This chapter recognises the importance of evaluation within housing for the benefit of service users, to support evidence-based occupational therapy practice within this setting and to promote continuous improvement of the overall service. The complexity of evaluating occupational performance within the home is analysed to encourage comprehensive evaluations to be undertaken. The chapter will help the reader to understand the competing demands for different types of information and enable them to make informed decisions related to the evaluation process. The importance of maintaining occupational therapy values while undertaking evaluation is emphasised. Both the process of service delivery and the outcomes of the service are identified as important areas to evaluate at two levels: those of the overall service and the individual service user. Two aspects of evaluation are explored in greater depth: the process of selecting appropriate outcome measures and a benchmarking initiative aimed at promoting best practice.

Introduction

Adaptations have a major impact on people's homes and family life and often involve undergoing a lengthy, complicated process to acquire. It is not sufficient to assume that thorough assessment, sound clinical reasoning and clear communication between all parties involved will be enough to assure quality service outcomes. Evaluation is also needed as the crucial final stage in the problem-solving process, without which there would be no possibility of reviewing either the achievement of individual goals or the standard of services. Without evaluation, old mistakes would be repeated and the frustration experienced by service users undergoing the process, or living with unsatisfactory adaptations, would continue. Equally, there would be no opportunity to learn from successful adaptations and examples of good practice or to work towards continuous improvement.

Within housing, OTs are responsible for recommending adaptations which require high levels of public spending and face ever-increasing demands for their service. They, therefore, need to undertake evaluation to justify this share of the public purse and to develop service efficiency and quality. There are three main drivers for occupational therapists to be actively involved in evaluation within housing. These are:

- the public sector emphasis on the effective and efficient use of public money to deliver quality services in an accountable manner;
- OTs have a professional responsibility to evaluate their services to safeguard good standards of practice (Creek, 2003), engage in evidence-based practice and continual professional development;
- disability rights and the rising expectations of the electorate (including both present and prospective service users).

Complexity of evaluating intervention in housing

Having recognised that it is essential to undertake evaluation, it should also be acknowledged that this is rarely a simple process within housing. The following two hypothetical case studies compare a relatively straightforward case with a more complex one and identify factors which influence the complexity of the evaluation process.

Case study 9.1
Mrs Giles is a 76-year-old lady who lives alone in a bungalow. She is in good health apart from osteoarthritis in her knees. Her only concern is difficulty sitting down safely onto her toilet since her towel rail has become loose as she had been using it to hold onto. She declined a raised toilet seat but agreed that a grab rail beside the toilet would be both useful and acceptable to her.

The evaluation process would be relatively straightforward because:

- a single occupational goal was identified – maintaining independence in toileting;
- only need to consider one person's perspective;
- the intervention would only have a minor impact on the home;
- relatively few people would be involved in service provision;
- it would be completed in a relatively short period of time;
- her functional ability is consistent.

Case study 9.2
Marina Sinclair is a 42-year-old wife and mother of three who has MS and has started to use her wheelchair in their home occasionally. They live in

a terraced house which has limited space for full wheelchair mobility. After detailed consultation, Marina decided to apply for a Disabled Facilities Grant (DFG) for a vertical lift and alterations to the ground floor to improve access into the house and around the kitchen and to provide a toilet and level-access shower.

The evaluation process would be more complex in this scenario because:

- the occupational goals identified would be more extensive, including those undertaken in her role as mother and wife as well as her own self-care needs;
- of the need to evaluate from the perspective of the whole family;
- the adaptations would have a major impact on the family home;
- the process will be complex and involve inter-agency working;
- the adaptations will take longer to complete;
- Marina has a degenerative condition and her functional ability fluctuates.

Evaluation should try to anticipate what future needs may be and how these may be met.

The following analysis, based on experience, aims to identify a range of factors which contribute to the complexity of evaluating intervention in housing. This level of understanding will help to ensure that an oversimplified process of evaluation is not adopted in practice.

Complexity of occupations

The first factor is the complex nature of occupations, which remain the primary focus for OTs in all settings. It is challenging to evaluate complex human activities within their environment in a way that can be easily communicated to others (Chard, 2004).

Goals for intervention

Evaluation methods selected should reflect the broad range of goals set within housing. It is inadequate to focus on a limited number of goals, such as improved levels of independence, especially when working with service users who have degenerative or life-limiting conditions.

The meaning of home

Housing adaptations can result in major, long-lasting changes to people's homes which have significance to individuals and family life. This is an extremely important area for service users and should not be excluded from the evaluation process.

Variety in housing

People live in a diverse range of home environments. The physical environment has a major impact on people's ability to carry out occupations within their home, and evaluation methods should take account of this inter-relationship.

Timing

Intervention in housing often takes a relatively long time to complete and has long-term effects. Therefore, the need for ongoing monitoring throughout the process and the appropriate timing of final evaluation must both be considered. If adaptations are evaluated before the builder is paid, then any immediate problems can be rapidly resolved, but this should be balanced with a system to appraise the longer-term effects of living with adaptations.

Large caseloads

Occupational therapists often carry very high caseloads with expectations for an immediate response. Consequently, owing to time pressure, there is a risk of OTs prioritising rapid assessment and intervention at the expense of sound clinical reasoning and evaluation.

Funding arrangements

The funding arrangements at both central and local levels often limit what can be recommended, which can, in turn, limit the effectiveness of outcomes. Evaluation methods should include a measure of unmet need and recognise that the option chosen may only partially meet the service user's preferences, owing to restrictions in funding.

Joint working

Good-quality adaptations require inter-professional and multi-agency working and often occur within the broader context of social care. This can result in a lack of clear attribution during evaluation and the tendency to deny responsibility when weaknesses are highlighted. The variation in style of service delivery also means that OTs are not always directly involved in the provision of services. In these situations joint working is needed during the evaluation process to encourage mutual responsibility to improve the overall service for the service user.

Political arena

There is a high demand for the service which is often disproportionate to the resources available and also political pressure from both central and local government to be accountable and demonstrate service standards. In this situation evaluation of efficient throughput and effective outcomes are both required.

Differing perspectives of quality and evaluation

Having explored the complexity of evaluation, the following section will revisit the reasons why evaluation is undertaken and analyse them in greater depth. This analysis aims to enable the reader to recognise the diverse and potentially conflicting uses of evaluation which exist within housing where differing types of information are required for divergent purposes.

The three main drivers for evaluation have been identified as: the legislative and managerial factors within the public sector, the professional imperatives of OT and disability rights and demands from the general public. These stakeholders are all interested in evaluating and improving the quality of the service. While this may initially appear to be a unified aim, the adoption of a more critical socio-political approach would suggest that quality should be understood as a social construct.

> Quality, much as beauty, can be seen to exist in the eye of the beholder, as different people experience it in different ways. (Pengelly, 1997, p. 14)

This raises the potential for separate agendas under the apparently unifying concept of the pursuit of quality (Wilkinson and Willmott, 1995). Rather than applying a unitary model, it is important to recognise the pluralist nature of quality and evaluation methods.

Public sector

Demographic changes, increased expectations and demands for adaptation services, combined with concurrent budget restraints, have resulted in governmental drives to restrain budget growth while simultaneously raising standards by making services more responsive to service users.

The challenge for government at both central and local levels is to reduce inputs while simultaneously improving outputs. Both require objective evaluation of the efficiency of the service (in terms of gaining the greatest output for the least resources) and the overall effectiveness of adaptations (in meeting expectations of government and the electorate).

The development and monitoring of performance standards also need to be understood in the political context of the ongoing power struggle between central and local government, where issues of respective responsibilities, provision of financial resources and issues around accountability are ongoing. Local government argues consistently for increased responsibility and funding to be devolved from the centre, while central government wants reassurance that the significant resources provided to local government have the desired impact for service users and offer value for money.

Local government managers within the organisation are responsible for delivering quality services at the operational level. They need evaluation methods which can demonstrate that the needs of the local population are being met effectively and within budget, based on the locally established policies and service standards, and which help them plan for the future development of services.

Occupational therapy

Beyond government and management directives it is also acknowledged good professional practice to measure the results of intervention and judge their effectiveness in order to be able to state the benefits of OT intervention and move towards improvement of service provision (COT, 2001a). Without evaluation, there is a greater risk of OTs being open to criticism from service users and the inspectorate, which would be inimical to the reputaion of the OT profession.

For practitioners, evaluation focuses upon measuring the effectiveness of the intervention for individuals, including the extent to which the adaptation has enabled them to engage in valued occupations. From a professional perspective, evaluation should be congruent with OT values (Hèrbert et al., 2000), which would mean evaluating from the client's perspective.

At a broader professional level, OTs have a responsibility to contribute to the continuing development of the profession through critical evaluation (COT, 2005). At the present time the use of outcome measures to evaluate OT service is recognised to be one of the most important factors underpinning evidence-based occupational therapy practice (Law et al., 2001).

Disability rights and service users

Individual service users and carers largely evaluate adaptations in terms of their subjective satisfaction with the process undertaken and the ongoing outcomes of living within their home following intervention. Much of this will link to the extent they felt involved in the decision-making process and how the adaptations have impacted upon family life and the meaning of their homes. For potential future service users the most relevant evaluation information will include waiting times and issues around equity. From a social model perspective, evaluation focuses on the extent to which the whole range of barriers have been removed.

Potential conflict

Having identified the range of differing perspectives and purposes for evaluation, the potential for conflict is evident. OTs within the setting will recognise that they sometimes feel caught between the political and managerial drives for efficiency and the client's idea of what constitutes a fully effective adaptation or more accessible service. From a disability-rights perspective, Oliver (1999) offers professionals a polarised choice between siding with disabled people or management. Abberley (2004) argued that OTs use the evaluation process to demonstrate the success of their intervention in order to validate their own work and drew attention to the potential conflict of interest in the providers of services also being the evaluators.

Once OTs recognise the diverse and potentially conflicting uses of evaluation and acknowledge the dilemmas under which they work, then they will be better equipped to make informed decisions about evaluation. This often involves balancing competing demands, for example ensuring that their evaluation methods measure both the efficiency of the service and the effectiveness of outcomes from the perspective of the service user. While recognising the importance of a balanced approach, it should be re-emphasised that this should not be at the expense of commitment to professional values. Organisational pressures to provide objective information about the effectiveness of the service, high levels of throughput and lower waiting lists should not overrule the commitment to maintaining a client-centred focus during evaluation and clearly identifying unmet need (COT, 2005).

Types of evaluation

There are two main areas which require evaluation for any service: first of all, how the service is delivered (process) and, secondly, the results of that service (outcome). Within housing, these need to be investigated on two different levels, that of the individual service user and of the overall service. Table 9.1 indicates the type of questions evaluation would seek to answer in relation to these.

Table 9.1 Types of evaluation

Area for evaluation	Individual service user	Overall service
Process	Was the adaptation completed correctly in reasonable time?	Are adaptations completed in a timely, efficient manner?
	Was there full consultation with the service user?	Are all standards being met?
		How can the service be improved?
Outcomes	Were they satisfied with all parts of the service? Did the adaptations enable the client to achieve their individual goals?	Are adaptations effective at enabling people to live independently within their own home?
	Were they and their family satisfied with the end result? Is further input required?	Are service users generally satisfied with their adaptations?

In order to provide information to answer this broad range of questions the evaluation process needs to be able to collect both quantitative and qualitative data. Quantitative, objective data are usually gathered by measuring service process against established standards and outcomes through the use of standardised outcome measures. In contrast, qualitative data collection methods aim to measure the subjective experience and perceptions of service users of both the delivery of the service and the final outcome of living with adaptations. Both are needed to provide a comprehensive evaluation.

A brief consideration of how the process of service delivery is measured demonstrates that these data collection methods can be effectively combined and that evaluation at the individual and service level is inter-related. In the past, process was evaluated mainly from the perspective of the service provider, focusing on waiting times, meeting criteria and following established procedures. The focus has now shifted towards also understanding how the process is experienced by service users (Heywood, 2001) including the extent to which they were valued and treated with respect (Heaton and Bamford, 2001). While the evaluation of individual service users is often based on qualitative measures to gain their opinions through interview, questionnaires or focus groups, this information can contribute towards the development of service standards and good-practice guides which provide reference points from which to collect quantitative data about the overall service. From these the process of continuous improvement can be undertaken.

The following sections of the chapter will explore two specific areas of evaluation in greater depth:

- the process of selecting appropriate outcome measures for use with individual service users;
- a benchmarking initiative aimed at promoting best practice and continuous improvement across the overall service.

Measuring outcomes for service users

Evaluation is the necessary final stage of the problem-solving process for OTs working with individual service users in any setting and is essential in housing, where adaptations have a major impact on people's homes and family life. Outcome measures are useful tools for OTs to use in this process because they record change over time, with an initial baseline being established prior to intervention and a reassessment being carried out once it has been completed (COT, 2001a).

Historical developments

An historical overview of the development of outcome measures to evaluate health showed that these have reflected the changing view of health and disability, moving from the former prevailing medical model towards a broader concept of quality of life (Bowling, 1997, 2001; McDowell and Newell, 1996). This is set out below:

- initial biomechanical focus based on survival rates and symptom relief;
- activities of daily living (ADL) scales measuring physical functioning in areas of mobility and self-care for use with people with high levels of dependency living in institutions;
- instrumental ADL (IADL) scales which also considered tasks necessary for living independently in the community such as shopping, preparing meals, doing housework and managing money;
- measures of social health and psychological well-being, including life satisfaction;
- broader measures of quality of life aimed to gain an overview of the global health, functioning and well-being of people.

The International Classification of Functioning, Disability and Health, or ICF, (WHO, 2001) encapsulates a broad view of health and embodies the shift of focus from disease towards activities and participation, which provides a theoretical basis for evaluation consistent with OT perspectives (Law et al., 2001).

An historical perspective also reveals a shift in the power relationship between professionals and disabled people with a move away from considering professionals to be the best qualified to measure all outcomes towards the increasing development of a more service-user-led measurement.

Outcome measurement within occupational therapy

It is important that the way OTs evaluate outcomes is consistent with their professional values. As a profession, occupational therapy has moved beyond a reductionist focus, with the accompanying measurement of component skills, towards an increasingly holistic approach to evaluation, which is more consistent with both its philosophy and the broad range of intervention goals aimed at improving quality of life (Liddle and McKenna, 2000). There is also an increased confidence within the profession to focus on occupational performance throughout the whole OT process.

Models of OT practice emphasise the need to consider the inter-relationship between the person, their environment and their occupations when evaluating occupational performance. One concept which is important to OTs working in housing is that of *environmental fit*, where a good fit enables the person to carry out their occupations to the best of their ability, while a poor fit would have a negative effect on their occupational performance (Law et al., 2001).

Historically, OTs have studied the person, the environment and the occupation as three distinct areas, with each contributing separately to the outcome of occupational performance. Standardised tools were used to measure the attributes of the person, activity analysis was used to examine occupations and observation checklists were used to measure the environment. OTs are now increasingly moving towards developing outcome measures which measure the interface between these areas (Law et al., 2001).

OTs are also aware of the importance of considering power relationships, and Law et al. (2001) have clearly identified the implications that client-centred occupational therapy practice have for evaluation. These include focusing evaluation on occupational performance issues identified by the client and ensuring that they have their say in evaluating the outcomes of therapy intervention.

Identification of outcomes

It is important to define expected outcomes before attempting to select measurement tools. While some interventions within housing are expected to result in improvement in function, others have alternative aims including maintenance at home, improved participation in the community or prevention of accidents. For example, when working with a client who has a degenerative neurological condition, the measurement of goal attainment in terms of their satisfaction and reduction of risk or carer strain may be more suitable goals than improvement in function. It is, therefore, important to identify clear goals relevant for individual clients, which can include both subjective experience and observable performance. These could include:

- achievement of client's and/or carer's occupational goals;
- eased access around the home/removal of physical barriers;
- maintaining family roles;
- improvement in function or increased independence;
- improvement in health or quality of life;
- increased safety/reduced risk of falls;
- reduced stress or risk of injury to carer;
- stay living at home;
- enhanced choice and control;
- increased privacy/dignity;
- client/carer satisfaction;
- increased social inclusion.

While it is vital to measure the anticipated outcomes, it is also useful to carry out a broader evaluation to identify unforeseen impacts of adaptation work which could be either positive or negative. For example, heating originally installed to increase independence in self-care following frequent epileptic fits may have the unanticipated impacts of reducing the number of fits experienced and improving family relationships. Alternatively, the installation of a vertical lift may have achieved increased levels of functional independence and safety but at the expense of some space in a family room.

Measuring outcomes

Having identified a range of potential outcomes from housing intervention, it is now necessary to consider how those outcomes can be measured. While the search for the single Holy Grail of outcome measures continues (Stubbs et al., 2004; Heaton and Bamford, 2001), the complexity of intervention within housing, and the diverse purposes for which the data are needed, make this an unrealistic quest. In practice more than one measure is often needed to gain a comprehensive picture.

This can be illustrated with reference to the two case studies considered earlier in this chapter. The selection of outcome measures is based on a clear understanding of the goals for the intervention with the specific individuals.

Case study 9.1 – revisited
Mrs Giles, the 76-year-old lady who lived alone in a bungalow and had osteoarthritis, had a grab rail installed to overcome her difficulty with toilet transfers.

The OT working with Mrs Giles could have measured goal attainment to assess the degree to which her individualised intervention goals had been attained. The process followed would have been to:

- identify the client's priorities;
- plan together specific and measurable goals;
- specify time for the measurement of goals;
- review goal attainment.

However, there is also a range of standardised outcome measures which could have been used to evaluate a variety of outcomes. As this intervention was aimed to improve her functional independence in ADL within her home, one of the following measures could have been used:

- *Community Dependency Index (CDI)* was developed in the United Kingdom to identify clients with a potential for increasing independence in self-care following environmental adaptation and to evaluate the outcome of this intervention for disabled and elderly people living in the community (Eakin and Baird, 1995).
- *Functional Independence Measure (FIM)* was designed in America to measure changes in functional ability and is now used internationally (McDowell and Newell, 1996). Within housing this could be used with the Enviro-FIM, which was designed to assess the influence of architectural design on functional performance including specific ADL tasks which involve physical access within the home (Danford and Steinfeld, 1997, cited in Law et al., 2001, p. 243).

As the intervention also sought to ensure that Mrs Giles could live safely at home with a reduced risk of her falling, the following could also be used:

- *Safety Assessment of Function and the Environment for Rehabilitation (SAFER)* was developed to evaluate the ability of older people to manage safely within their own home focusing on ADL and IADL within the physical home environment (Community Occupational Therapists and Associates, 1991, cited in Letts et al., 1998, p. 127);
- *Falls Efficacy Scale* was used to measure a client's confidence in carrying out ADL without falling on a scale 1–3 which could be used to measure change in confidence before and after intervention (Tinnetti et al., 1990);

- *Westmead Home Safety Assessment* was published in Australia and used to identify fall hazards in the homes of older adults based on a comprehensive literature review (Clemson, 1997, cited in Law et al., 2001, p. 239).

Evaluation of a more complex case may require the use of a broader range of outcome measures.

> **Case study 9.2 – revisited**
> Marina Sinclair, the 42-year-old wife and mother with MS, had a DFG for a vertical lift and alterations to the ground floor to improve access to the house, alter the kitchen and provide an accessible toilet and shower.

As there were many potential goals to focus on during this intervention, the OT could have chosen to identify Marina's priorities by using the:

- *Canadian Occupational Performance Measure (COPM)*: an individualised measure designed to record change in a client's self-perception of, and satisfaction with, their occupational performance over time (Law et al., 1994). It ensures client-centred practice by focusing on occupational performance areas of importance to the individual.

As part of the purpose of the intervention was to maintain her independence in ADL through the modification of the home environment, it would be useful to measure these aspects using:

- *The Housing Enabler*: a detailed tool developed in Sweden to measure the inter-relationship between the functional limitations of an individual and their housing environment from which an accessibility score is calculated which represents the combination of both the functional problems of the individual and the physical barriers in their housing (Iwarsson, 1999).

As functional independence is not the only purpose of the intervention it would be useful to measure the other aspects which could include Marina's perception of her social inclusion using:

- *Community Integration Measure*: a brief client-centred measure using a research-based definition of integration, initially developed for use with people with brain injury, now used more widely (McColl and Davies, 1998, cited in Law et al., 2001, p. 220).

As this intervention affected other family members it would also be important to measure its impact upon them, including stress levels of the husband as carer:

- *Caregiver Strain Index:* a measure to identify the strain experienced by carers including sleep disturbance, financial pressures and competing demands on time (Robinson, 1983). It was initially developed for use with carers of physically impaired elderly people living at home, but has since been used with carers across all age ranges (Stewart and Neyerlin-Beale, 2000).

Consideration of these two case studies has demonstrated that there is no single outcome measurement which will be suitable to evaluate all housing interventions with every client. Most standardised outcome measures tend to focus on single aspects of a complex picture, making it important not to use them in isolation but as component parts of a comprehensive evaluation process. The ICF has been suggested as an integrative framework within which to do this. McDonald et al. (2004) used it to organise a range of outcome measures to evaluate seating interventions at home with children with cerebral palsy. This included *impairment* (e.g. reduction of deformity/pain), *activities* (ability to play/write from stable sitting position) and *participation* (involvement in family interaction/meals) within the child's environmental context. Alternatively, a model of OT practice can be used to select a comprehensive range of outcome measures (Law et al., 2001).

A review of the literature on evaluation methods used in practice showed that OTs prefer to develop tools locally rather than use existing outcome measures (Heaton and Bamford, 2001). However, it is worth checking what is already available as the effort involved in developing a measure should not be underestimated. Good-quality outcome measures need to be rigorously tested for reliability and validity, and the development of a standardised measure requires several years of extensive research (COT, 2001a).

Another temptation is to alter existing outcome measures to fit local demands, or use them with a different client group or within a different setting from that for which they were designed. However, if this is done, it should be recognised that the previous work on reliability and validity is no longer applicable. As outcome measures have been developed internationally it is also important to consider whether they have been validated for use within the user's own country, for example the Housing Enabler was initially validated for use in Sweden as it was based on Swedish accessible housing standards.

There is a broad range of existing outcome measures available to OTs working within housing, and their effective use requires a clear understanding of the purpose for which the measure was developed to prevent them from being used for incompatible reasons. This was demonstrated by Stubbs et al. (2004), who report that the CDI had not met their expectations, which had been to reflect the complexity and diversity of the presenting problems faced by OTs within the Social Services team. This was not surprising, as the primary purpose of the CDI was as a focused tool to target resources towards services which promoted independence (Eakin and Baird, 1995). Stubbs et al. (2004) recognised that quality of life measures were more appropriate for measuring the breadth of outcomes from their practice and that the CDI could usefully be used alongside these to specifically measure changes in ADLs within the home.

To help with the selection of outcome measures, the use of information packs (COT, 2001a) and critical reviews (Law et al., 2001) is invaluable. Both sources of information will state the purpose of each listed outcome measure and provide information about where it can be obtained and suggestions for further reading. A critical review will also evaluate its reliability, validity and its strengths and weaknesses for use in practice. As the development of outcome measures is ongoing, it is important to be aware of and refer to the most up-to-date information available.

While the focus of this section has been on the selection of outcome measures for use with individual service users, it should be recognised that they can also be used to evaluate the overall service. Stewart and Neyerlin-Beale (2000) used COPM, CDI and carer strain scales to investigate the effectiveness of paediatric occupational therapy within Social Services. They argue that the combination of subjective user-controlled evaluation tools, such as COPM, and objective information from the CDI could provide managers with a comprehensive evaluation of OT provision in Social Services. Johnson (1998) cited in Awang (2004) also suggests that COPM is an effective measure which can be used alongside other community care measures.

Measuring service performance

OT housing work does not happen simply in isolated episodes but as part of an overall service. The organisation from which the OT operates will be considering not simply whether a specific case has been satisfactorily completed but also how this case relates to all the other cases the service deals with. It is important to give individual episodes a context by measuring against expected standards of service delivery. By doing this it is possible to measure overall performance of the service, to judge whether the standards of service are being met, to identify service process or resource issues as they arise and to help to plan future service delivery.

Effective evaluation of the overall service should include a detailed examination of the existing service to enable the establishment of clear aims for future development. While there are many evaluation tools which can be used in this process, including audit and system review, this section will focus on benchmarking and the development of service standards drawing on the work of the Syniad Benchmarking Centre based in Wales.

Benchmarking housing adaptations

In order to understand this benchmarking initiative it is important to understand the political context in which it was developed. During the 1980s in the UK, central government attempted to direct local government towards the business approaches used by the private sector. This reached its apogee with the programme of Compulsory Competitive Tendering (CCT), where local authority services were required to be exposed to competitive tendering with private sector providers, within defined quality parameters.

With the election of the Labour Government in 1997, there was pressure from local government on the incoming administration to discard CCT, which was widely disliked. The challenge for the new Government was to introduce an alternative form of public-sector accountability that would be more acceptable for local government but would provide a means of holding local government to account.

The framework introduced was Best Value, which incorporated the principles of balancing service quality and cost. This required all local authority services to be exposed to Best Value Service Review over a five-year period. These intensive reviews were criticised for wasting resources where there may already be evidence that services were demonstrably performing well.

This led to a review and the development of new models. In England this was called the Comprehensive Performance Review (CPR) and depended on a collation of audit and inspection data to provide an opinion of the service ranging from 'poor', 'weak', 'fair', 'good' to 'excellent'.

In Wales quite a different framework emerged called the Wales Programme for Improvement (WPI). This reflected the changes brought about by devolution in 1997, since the inception of Best Value and the creation of the Welsh Assembly Government. It was assisted by having 22 unitary authorities in Wales, created through local government reorganisation in 1996. WPI took a different tack to the English model by requiring Welsh local government to self-assess their overall performance leading to the production of an Action Plan. This Action Plan and self-assessment was validated by external audit.

These developments highlighted a continuing tension between central and local government relating to responsibility for service delivery and accountability. They also demonstrated the noticeable establishment of the principles and practices of performance management.

Performance management was well established in the private sector but was comparatively new for local government and presented considerable challenges for managers and practitioners to understand and apply. This was especially so due to the diverse nature of local authority services, which aim to meet wide-ranging needs while operating within complex service environments.

Housing and adaptations were identified as being among the central services required to sustain independent living in the community (Welsh Office, 1996). It was also recognised that co-operative service working within authorities was essential, for example between housing and social care, especially where different functions relating to adaptations were carried out by different departments. Close co-ordination between those departments, and between individuals within the departments, was recommended (Welsh Office, 1978).

While it was recognised that agencies involved in housing adaptations work needed to work together to plan strategically, allocate resources and deliver a combined service, this was frequently difficult to achieve in practice. The wholesale reorganisation of local government in Wales in 1996 provided a significant opportunity for a more effective co-ordination of the planning and delivery of services to people with disabilities, by combining former housing and welfare authorities into single-tier unitary authorities.

Performance comparisons

With this backdrop, a benchmarking club was established in 1999 with the support of Care & Repair Cymru and the Welsh Assembly Government. The club comprised 19 of the 22 Welsh unitary authorities. The Syniad Benchmarking Centre, located within the Improvement and Development arm of the Welsh Local Government Association, co-ordinated and facilitated the benchmarking study.

Benchmarking

Benchmarking is an evaluation tool used within performance management. It takes its name from a surveying benchmark, which is a reference point, a constant against which measurements and comparisons can be made. This definition is fundamental to understanding benchmarking, which involves the establishment of a reference point from which comparisons can be made. It is a technique which takes a comprehensive view of cost, quality, delivery systems and customer satisfaction and can be applied to secure improvements in virtually any setting across all sectors. Benchmarking can be described as a process of striving for levels of excellence in performance through systematically comparing performance and processes between and within organisations (CIPFA, 1996). This drive for continuous improvement is based on learning how to do things better.

The Welsh Assembly Government recognised that the potential for learning from service performance comparison was maximised when they were used to identify and seek an explanation for differences which in turn could inform decisions on future improvements (Great Britain 1996, Welsh Assembly Government, 2000).

The work of the benchmarking study was to examine the service of housing adaptations, within which, although recognised as an area for which significant government guidance exists, considerable variation occurs in the structure, organisation and delivery of the service. In particular it was recognised from the outset that there was significant variation in the time taken for the process from enquiry/referral to completion of adaptation works. This variability in practice standards was an area the club was keen to address in order that practice standards might be developed and recommended for national application, resulting in a greater degree of future service consistency.

The study sought to develop valid performance measures and systems through:

- gathering detailed comparative information from participating authorities;
- devising Good Practice Guides for agreed areas of the service;
- devising robust and appropriate performance indicators to measure subsequent performance.

The benchmarking approach adopted was to develop a service profile of the entire function, taking into account resources, staff numbers, grades of staff, ICT systems, use of time-recording systems, service policies, partnership working, monitoring procedures etc. In addition the club determined to focus upon four core areas of the service:

- communications;
- needs assessment/prioritisation/eligibility;
- time taken;
- service outcome.

Once the subject had been determined, and the scope and parameters confirmed, the club was able to move onto the phase of data gathering and analysis. This began with an assessment of existing data including that from the Audit Commission, the Welsh Assembly Government and the DoH. At this point the club confirmed that there was a data gap between the data which already existed and that which would be required. Detailed data question-naires were developed to bridge this gap, which required completion by different service departments, in each local authority, including Social Services and Housing for the financial year 1998/99.

Principal study findings

The study confirmed the complexity of the housing adaptations service, the existence of the varied interpretations of the legislation and different funding routes which resulted in services which had not always been readily accessible to service users and had varied in their consistency.

Key findings included:

- The complexity of the adaptations service meant that access by clients was not generally well understood. A number of authorities in Wales had attempted to address this through restructuring to provide a dedicated adaptations service using a 'whole systems' approach.
- Local authorities had notable difficulty in providing data relating to the time taken from enquiry to the completion of works. As this was seen as a crucial performance dimension of the adaptations service it was recommended that the club gave consideration to developing a model which detailed the key stages of the service process against which target times would be set and performance measured.
- Inequalities in the arrangements for providing housing adaptations, which varied across tenure and between authorities, resulted in some service users being disadvantaged by virtue of their geographical location. It was recommended that consideration should be given to consolidating all forms of funding allocated for housing adaptations and to the development of clear service eligibility criteria, common practice standards and times for process completion.
- All authorities in the benchmarking club had a process for prioritising referrals with most using three levels of priority. It was recommended that a standard priority system could be adopted across Welsh local government.
- While most authorities had tracking systems in place to monitor the progress of applications, few had cross-service departmental arrangements. It was recommended that Welsh local government gave consideration to developing cross-service tracking systems to monitor the progress of applications thereby gathering performance data on the time undertaken for the entire process.
- There was a variety of 'fast-track' routes, mainly used for minor adaptations. It was recommended that the benchmarking club gave consideration to developing fast-track systems with established eligibility criteria and forms of speedy options analysis.

Overall, the report highlighted the complexity of service provision by different local authority departments and external agencies and the confusion that this can present to service users. This complexity meant that performance measurement was rarely integrated – this being highlighted by the significant lack of performance data for the time taken in measuring the entire process. Some processes were measured, but these were not fully integrated into the performance measurement of the overall process. It was recommended that the club, in association with the Welsh Assembly Government, consider this issue further with a view to devising models of performance measurement to include:

* time of process;
* effectiveness of tracking systems for monitoring;
* systems for providing information to clients;
* systems for evaluation of service quality;
* systems for needs assessment, prioritisation and eligibility;
* systems for signposting clients to appropriate services.

Developing service standards

Performance management in local government is moving away from performance targets to performance standards. In Wales this has been undertaken through the development of practice standards in the form of Good Practice Guides (GPGs).

In the field of housing adaptations GPGs were developed in the following five areas (SBC, 2001):

* Screening for Eligibility and Prioritisation for Assessment;
* Adaptation Needs Assessment;
* Time Taken;
* Ensuring a Quality Outcome;
* Ensure an Effective Communication Process.

The GPGs were designed to enable these service areas to establish Minimum Standards, to assess their current performance in comparison with others and to set goals for future improvement.

The intention with GPGs is that all authorities should at least be achieving Minimum Standards – these were carefully pitched at a level conceived to be reasonable and practicable for authorities to achieve. This is an important professional point as the practical application of GPGs

Table 9.2 Standards within Good Practice Guides

Key activity	Minimum practice	Good practice	Better practice
Elements 1, 2, 3 ... etc.	What you should be doing now	What some are doing now and all should aim for	What 'best in class' services are achieving

would mean that services not achieving Minimum Standards would be regarded as underperforming/failing.

Table 9.3 Example from Good Practice Guide

Key activity	Minimum practice	Good practice	Better practice
7. Funding arrangements	Service user advised of possible alternative sources of funding	Regular budget meetings to ensure clear understanding of budget availability/restraints Regular meetings between professionals to review expenditure Financial targets in place for professionals	Joint commissioning/ shared budgets to maximise resources effectively All staff to be aware of financial management principles and training provided if necessary

In addition to Minimum Standards, the Guides set out Good Practice and Better Practice standards. Local authority services should aim to achieve a performance balance within this practice standards matrix.

The following example is taken from the fifth GPG (SBC, 2001), focusing on effective communication, and uses the key activity of communication related to funding to illustrate how the standards operate.

GPGs serve as guidance on the standards to be attained in service provision. Beyond setting Minimum Standards, it is for individual authorities to determine what service standards they provide. Such determinations should take account of local needs, priorities and available resources and be consistent with the requirements of the local authority strategic and performance planning processes, as contained in their Performance/ Business/Community Plans.

Beyond the three levels of practice standards contained in the GPGs, there are also included critical success factors (CSFs), being the elements that are required to be in place to provide a good-quality service and the criteria against which the organisation can be judged. They are the equivalent of high-level service objectives and can be regarded as the characteristics of a successful service.

Defining CSFs is a relatively simple but powerful exercise that focuses questions on what service professionals do, why they do it and whether they should be doing it. This will often provoke professionals with a welcome challenge to think about the service they provide and what purpose it serves/should serve.

The GPGs are intended to be live, working documents whose content is likely to alter over time, reflecting changes in what is regarded as good and better practice. They are not prescriptive but serve to help service practitioners understand their current performance position and to think through where they wish to move the service to better respond to need.

The benefits of using GPGs can include the following:

- set Minimum Standards (if these do not already exist);
- provide a structured framework to understand current performance levels and to plan service improvements;
- assist teams to focus on service areas where effort should be concentrated;
- reinforce the principles of objective setting and performance management;
- facilitate and complement the technique of benchmarking;
- encourage the sharing of expertise and good practice and promote the comparison of service performance with other providers.

This section has described work conducted in Wales to benchmark the housing adaptations service. The findings of this work confirmed that significant service variations occurred in the delivery of this service and, as part of the working approach, service standards were developed in the form of GPGs. This pre-empted the introduction of performance management principles into Social Services (Social Services Inspectorate Wales, 2001) and helped Welsh local authorities to develop forms of accountability, which were developed by service professionals and were satisfactory for the accountability requirements of central government. The GPGs established minimum service standards that were developed by service professionals for their professional peers. They provided a unique service perspective, offering a framework for services to select service standards and set appropriate service objectives, with the flexibility for adaptation to meet local circumstances, needs and priorities. Finally, they encouraged the gathering of performance evidence to demonstrate whether the service was delivering on these targets.

This benchmarking study was always regarded as work in progress. Further work was begun in late 2003, supported by the Welsh Assembly Government and the Welsh Local Government Association, intended to build on the previous work. The areas being investigated are:

- needs assessment and prioritisation;
- integrated working practices;
- service equity.

A further six areas have been identified as elements of the service that would benefit from the development of Good Practice Guides, these are:

- provision of community equipment;
- Regulatory Reform Order – opportunities and good practice stemming from;
- occupational therapy staff – recruitment, retention and best use of;
- terminal illness and palliative care;
- services to children;
- relationships to Registered Social Landlords and partners.

It is expected that this phase of the study will be complete by November 2005. Further information and copies of the GPGs are available through the WLGA website, following the links to 'Improvement' and then 'Benchmarking'.

The evaluation of the overall service is important to:

- recognise the problems caused by service variation;
- develop service standards to deliver greater service consistency;
- recognise the need for performance measurement and verification against these standards;
- reinforce the principles of performance management and the benefits to be derived from this;
- provide mechanisms of accountability and opportunities for self-regulation.

Professionals, including OTs, need to be involved in the evaluation of the overall service at this level. This is important for central/local government relations and to re-establish confidence and trust so that the two can work together, in partnership, on the modernisation agenda of public service. More importantly, it will lead to the levelling out of current service inconsistencies and inequalities, promoting the continuous improvement of housing adaptations services.

Conclusion

Housing adaptations work has a major, long-term impact on people's home and family life. There is also an ever-increasing demand for this service, which requires extensive public investment. Within this context, housing services need to demonstrate that they can provide an efficient service, including effective outcomes and accountability. OTs working within housing have been challenged to use evaluation for the benefit of service users, to support evidence-based practice within OT in this setting and to promote the continuous improvement of the overall service.

This chapter has recognised the importance of evaluation to review whether goals have been achieved in an acceptable way with individual service users and to identify areas of service performance which require improvement. To enable this to happen it has sought to encourage occupational therapists to make conscious decisions about why they take part in the evaluation process, how appropriate data are best generated and how they will be used within an integrated system of evaluation to improve overall service provision.

While evaluation has been identified as being essential within housing, it has also been acknowledged to be a complex process requiring pragmatic as well as conceptual decisions. The following process is suggested to help make informed decisions when selecting evaluation methods in practice.

* Clarify why the evaluation is being carried out, how it fits with overall evaluation process and how it will be used to improve the service.
* Ascertain what needs to be evaluated (process/outcome/both) and at what level this needs to be measured (individual/service/both).
* Decide what type of information is required.
* Consider the advantages and disadvantages of using existing measurement tools (including standardised outcome measures and standards of practice).
* Consider if the methods suggested are acceptable to service users and congruent with OT values.
* Review available resources and consider how feasible this method of evaluation would be in practice (time consumption/ease of use/training required/when it would be carried out and by whom).
* Decide how the results will be recorded and communicated to others at all levels as it is important to incorporate them into the administrative system.
* Carry out the evaluation and use the information gathered to ensure effective intervention, provide evidence to support practice and establish goals for future improvements in service.

Key points

* Evaluation is the final stage of the problem-solving process, which is essential to providing an evidence base within housing services to ensure that appropriate and acceptable adaptations are provided efficiently and effectively.
* The major aim for evaluation is the improvement of services for service users.
* It is important to recognise the complexity of evaluation within housing to ensure that a comprehensive process is undertaken.
* Evaluation must be based on fully informed decisions as to why we take

part in the process and how the data will be used within an integrated system.

- Ensure congruence between occupational therapy values and the evaluation methods selected.
- Both process of service delivery and outcomes are important areas to evaluate for the individual service user and the overall service.
- Having investigated a range of evaluation tools, it is clear that no single one is sufficient: an integrated, comprehensive ongoing system of evaluation is required.
- Evaluation methods based on performance management can help provide consistent, accountable public services.
- There remains much scope for research and development in the area of evaluation in housing, including outcome measurement and management information systems.

CHAPTER 10

Smart technology at home

KATHRYN MCNAB

The future of housing design may look very different depending on the uptake and use of smart technology now in development. The technology was introduced in Chapter 1 as a codicil to the planning, design and building section and has great potential to influence the way that planning, design and construction work is undertaken as well as providing individualised personal support at home. Options for living at home may be radically increased when such systems are integrated into housing design.

Introduction

The aim of this chapter is to convey some of the fundamental skills and aims of practice employed by occupational therapists when using new technologies, while considering the principles and theories that underpin their use (Hagedorn, 2000). Experience gained by the author is based on work done in West Lothian Council in Scotland using smart technology in the community with the aim of assisting people to remain more safely in their own homes for longer. The process of experimentation with new and prototype technologies and the subsequent progression to a thriving mainstream service for older or vulnerable people living in their own homes will be used as a case study example and will be described throughout the chapter.

In this case study the origins and development of the project are described along with the rationale for change and the need for new models of care. Implementation issues and practical experiences including learning and feedback from the pilot process are given with case study examples of some of the earlier applications of technology. Explanations of the assessment processes and process for matching technology to needs are detailed and issues such as ethical dilemmas are considered, along with the importance of evaluation and review of interventions. The service continues to develop and future planning in smart housing is illustrated. The chapter concludes with some key messages for occupational therapists working in this field.

Background information to the case study project

Maintaining and supporting people at home is the aim of all government policies in Europe (Astrid Group, 2000). Changing demographic patterns and the high cost of providing institutional-based care have contributed to this shift towards community-based services. With the advent of the National Health Service and Community Care Act 1990 in the UK came new legislation placing the emphasis on Local Authority provisions in the community. For example, Modernising Community Care (Scottish Office, 1998) stressed the importance of caring for people, wherever possible, in their own home and, where found to be impossible, providing care within as domestic a scale environment as possible. There is, as a consequence, a renewed emphasis on the user and their quality of life, which reflects the holistic approach long favoured by occupational therapists, taught to see the person as an individual and to promote maximum functionality at home.

The Disability Rights Commission's mission is to achieve a society in which all disabled people can participate fully as equal citizens. Central to this is the right of disabled people to live independently, with choices, dignity and appropriate controls (Goodridge, 2004). At home it is easier to have control over one's own environment, where it is possible to be surrounded by personal possessions, choose the way of life, the routines adopted and to value the privacy afforded by this.

Bjornaby et al. (1999) found that making decisions and controlling our own lives is important for the majority of us. What does home mean to people? The old adage that 'There is no place like home' suggests that home is about security, safety, comfort, convenience, familiarity, personal space and possessions. Living at home means proximity to friends, family and other non-formal care and support mechanisms. Contact with people making deliveries, meter readers, doorstep traders or window cleaners may seem trivial on the surface but contribute to a vital and often overlooked network of social stimulation and sense of community and belonging in society. Most people prefer to be able to live in their own homes, and recent research would support this (Bowes and McColgan, 2005; Evans, 2003).

When people become disabled or frail due to advancing years, their situation at home may become more tenuous. Suddenly, the things they have done for years without needing to think about them become more difficult and as a result their safety, security, comfort and convenience – the things so much valued about being at home – are under threat (DoH, 2000b).

An exciting challenge therefore is to find ways to address the key issues of safety, security and comfort. This may be done by designing and equipping domestic housing so that people can confidently remain in the familiarity of their own home. The use of different types of technology can contribute to this process not only for the benefit of the person but also for the family and carers too as without the knowledge, skill or the vision they may not have confidence in the person's ability to remain safely at home (Judd, 1997). This often results in a conflict of interest, when the person wishes, despite the perceived risks, to remain at home and the relatives are concerned that they should be placed in a protected environment where they will be looked after and therefore assumed to be safe. Social workers and community occupational therapists frequently come across this conflict of interest, particularly in relation to the care of older people. It usually arises when informal carers are feeling the strain of juggling the caring role while carrying on with their own lives, and it often results in the person feeling under an obligation to agree to move into a care setting.

Occupational therapists working in the community to promote maximal independence often struggle with the dilemma of recommending care or continuing with possible personal and domestic activities, usually without the human or financial resources for rehabilitation. It could be argued that with the provision of packages of care dependency is encouraged. Often, care is provided because it is felt that carrying out certain tasks, such as using the cooker, increases the risk to the person. Alternatively, free choice may be disregarded with the cooker being disconnected or removed altogether. Were this to happen, it is not surprising if the person feels devalued or becomes accustomed to a carer going in every day to prepare a main meal. Once this type of service is underway, it is often in place for an indefinite period of time; so it could be argued that providing care increases dependency on others. Everything should be done to proactively preserve the choice, safety and independence of the individual, before more major decisions which will have a greater impact on the person are taken.

Risk management is a whole subject in itself and is explored in more detail in Chapter 8, but frequently occupational therapy intervention is about weighing up the risks and finding ways to reduce them while focusing on maximising independent living. Assessing risk is usually about negotiation and compromise in order to achieve a safe, efficient and positive outcome for clients and carers which minimises risks and is acceptable to all parties.

Life can never be risk free (something that relatives, in particular, find difficult to cope with), but technology has a role in helping to manage the risks while allowing the person to continue living life as normally as possible. Occupational therapists can contribute to this area, as demonstrated by this pilot of technology in the community. It was clear that there was definite potential to promote greater safety and independence within an environment where the risk was managed more effectively.

Establishment of the project

The initial stages of establishing this project show how the development of new services require a socio-political approach to secure agreement on the necessity for the new service among the organisations involved and resources to implement it (see 'Socio-political approaches', Chapter 1).

With the new Modernising Community Care (Scottish Office, 1998) legislation in place, West Lothian Council set out to provide a change in the patterns of care for the residents of its residential care homes for older people with support needs. In order to achieve this aim a detailed strategy was developed to extend the range of provision for older people needing support. The objective was to develop a design of house and system of support that would sustain independent living within a domestic environment.

A plan of this size and scope required co-operation between health, social care and housing organisations. In April 1998, the Joint West Lothian Plan for Services for Older People was agreed by the Primary and Community Care Planning partners, Lothian Health, West Lothian Council, West Lothian NHS Trust, the independent sector, users and carers. This partnership agreed that there would be a major move away from the provision of council residential care places (which were not guaranteed to meet new Care Standards), and instead there would be created more housing with care and very sheltered housing, linked with the development of a small number of specialist and high-quality residential units. The strategy aimed to offer a broad range of support from independent living through to services to individuals with high levels of dementia or physical dependency. A key element was to increase choice for older people and to move away from the continuum of care whereby, as their needs increased, people would move (often outside their own locality) into increasingly intensive care settings. Instead, the planned approach would be to deliver the care to meet needs where people chose to live (Bowes and McColgan, 2005).

The Local Authority aimed to use New Housing Partnership Funding via the Scottish Executive to develop a revolutionary range of provision for older people with support needs. It would utilise new forms of design and technology to enhance the independence and quality of life for older people needing support. The council acted as enabler, performing the project management role, arranging relocation and demolition, providing the land and some resources to their partners who then were to build and manage the new provision. The objective was to diversify the range of provision available to allow meaningful choices for older people in need of support. Additionally, the council received New Housing Partnership Funding for the piloting of Smart Technology.

Aims of the project

The aims were to provide the area with a support infrastructure which would:

- enable older people to live longer in their own homes, retaining their independence and self-value;
- set in place a model of care which would be provided in partnership with other providers such as housing associations and Scottish Homes;
- release funding which was tied up in institutional care, for investment in the development of community-based care, as required by government guidance;
- to be the basis of a wider strategic approach to the provision of services for older people;
- to diversify the tenure of home-based support from local authority to housing associations and provide access to new technologies at home for owner/occupiers;
- to attract a significant level of private finance;
- to reflect community need by providing services in locations where there is real need.
  (West Lothian Council, 1998)

Funding was secured for a four-year pilot project called the Opening Doors for Older People Project. This developed two different housing- based models utilising smart technology, Housing with Care Developments and the Smart Support at Home Service. The Smart Support at Home Service is nowadays a mainstreamed service known as the Home Safety Service.

More information on the various phases of the project including funding and cost analysis suggesting significant cost benefits of the new services can be found in the latest report from Bowes and McColgan (2005).

Housing with Care

The council's existing residential care facilities, while still meeting a need, were considered to offer an outdated (institutionalised) model of care.

Here, it seemed, was a golden opportunity to create more choice for older people. As it was not considered feasible to upgrade the existing homes, it was decided instead to demolish and rebuild with a new concept – Housing with Care developments. In managing these radical changes, a considerable amount of public liaison was required to explain and reassure that the closure of buildings, which were people's homes, would in the end provide a better alternative for the residents.

The fundamental principle of Housing with Care is that people should not be removed from their own communities when needing care; the staff, facilities and services such as shops should come to them. Each person is a tenant rather than a resident (so that they may receive housing benefit if applicable), having their own front door and complete domestic facilities within. Design specifications took into account the need to give special consideration to the needs of, for example, people with dementia. Each property was planned and built to the space standards of a two-apartment house, barrier free and suitable for varying degrees of mobility.

Housing with Care complexes may have 'land-marking' design features which incorporate or recreate things important to the local community. An example of this is a war memorial which is located at the entrance to one of the new complexes because of the community's preference that the memorial should remain on its original site. The developments have been designed on a streetscape idea with the 'hub' incorporating a village shop, café, hairdresser and community room with the idea being that members of the wider community use the facilities in the same way as the tenants, so maintaining and encouraging local communication and support networks. The objective is to create a domestic environment that supports the individual rather than an institutional environment, but also to be part of the community rather than just within the community. Each development consists of a cluster of buildings containing in the region of thirty houses with associated communal hub facilities, linked by a corridor and staff support areas. Each individual's tenancy is fitted with a core package of smart technology to enable emergency management and increase both personal and environmental safety and security. Housing with Care aims to maximise the support for people living at home and comprises a multi-skilled housing support team and new technology. Levels of service provision are much higher than the former residential care model and aim to provide a seamless service which is not typical of sheltered or extra-sheltered care schemes.

The Home Safety Service

The Home Safety Service follows the same core principles as Housing with Care, that is to increase both the support and protection for the individual and the retention and protection of the domestic environment. The Home Safety Service is provided by the Council's Health and Social Care Team and is directed to older people living in dispersed homes in the community where they may have resided for many years. However, people with physical disabilities, mental health problems and people vulnerable in other ways, for example due to domestic abuse or victims of crime, may also apply for the Home Safety Service. The Health and Social Care Team operates 365 days a year from 7am to 10pm and is also responsible for two other related services: Rapid Response and Rehabilitation in the Community.

The Home Safety Service can be applied for by the householder themselves or by a professional acting on their behalf. A core package of technology (see Table 10.1) is provided as standard, with a wide range of personal add-ons being prescribed as required on an assessed-need basis. The technology is supported by the multi-skilled staff of the Health and Social Care Team. Some people need additional support with the technology and so are allocated keyworkers from the team who maintain a regular contact. Others may need assistance in the event of an emergency,

Table 10.1 Core package of technology and potential add-on equipment

Core package based on social alarm technology	Lifeline home unit
	Pendant
	Smoke detector
	Temperature extremes sensor (heat and cold)
	2 flood detectors
	2 passive infrared movement detectors (inactivity and/or intruder)
Examples of add-on equipment	
Environmental sensors	Carbon monoxide or natural gas detectors
Wandering sensors	e.g. door contact with PIRs (passive infrared sensors), bed occupancy sensors
Medication reminders	e.g. voice prompts delivered via the home unit
Beacons, sounders, pagers	e.g. to alert those with sensory impairment that alarm triggered
Lifestyle monitoring sensors	Profiles the person's normal behaviour and alerts if deviance occurs
Video door entry	Enables the person to see and speak to the caller on the doorstep. Can be linked to the TV and remote door-release mechanism
Email and Internet technology	Increases range of social contacts and promotes independence e.g. with shopping
Environmental control equipment	Allows independent command of electrically powered devices within the home

NB. this list is not exhaustive and will change with the development of new technologies.

such as a flood or a fall. If they do not have relatives or friends locally to respond in an emergency, the team has two staff on call every night and is able to provide the appropriate assistance on a 24-hour basis.

The council had to decide how best to meet the considerable costs of providing such a service. It was debated at length whether or not to pass on some of the cost to the clients. Now, when a person applies for the Home Safety Service, they complete a financial assessment form which is forwarded to a benefits adviser (who does a benefits check and assists with income maximisation) and a calculation is made as to whether the applicant can afford the subsidised weekly charge (currently £4.87). This charge covers the loan of the equipment (there is no increase in cost to the client for additional equipment), 24-hour connection to the control centre, support as required from the Health and Care Team staff, engineer attendance, ongoing maintenance/upgrade and annual battery replacement and servicing.

At the outset, there were many questions about the application of technology in the domestic environment and in particular it was wondered how older people would cope with having it introduced into their homes. It was assumed that older people would be resistant to, or unable to cope with, this method of intervention. For an occupational therapist, the challenge was there to apply assessment skills with a view to finding and utilising some new solutions to situational problems.

Many people are daunted at the prospect of using technology. Before working on the Opening Doors for Older People Project, all staff had very limited or no knowledge about smart technology. Colleagues expressed fears about their own ability to understand, assess for and use new equipment. They also found it difficult to know whether it would be acceptable and usable with, for example, dementia sufferers. Concerns were voiced about the 'Big Brother' remote surveillance approach to monitoring the well-being of vulnerable older people and whether this was an ethical way forward. Issues relating to reliability, programming, servicing and maintenance were all raised. There were also anxieties concerning lack of knowledge, difficulties in understanding technical jargon and fears of apparent inadequacy when dealing with technical experts.

On the strategic side there was the dilemma of whether the specialist approach should be maintained or whether it would be preferable to aim to enable assessment and support staff across the board to develop the necessary skills to assess for technology solutions. It was felt that the latter option would require comprehensive training for staff and ongoing refresher training on a regular basis. It would also be more demanding than some staff would welcome.

A decision was taken to organise briefing sessions and workshops with assessment and support staff in order to establish a baseline of their views/concerns and introduce them to the concept of using technology. Application examples were given, along with the reassurance that they were only being asked to identify the need and consider whether technology could help, without having to have such expertise as to identify the solution. A workbook to aid learning and direct thinking was produced as well as an online learning support package. These training opportunities were favourably received and staff responded positively by making largely appropriate recommendations for further technology assessment.

Development of the project

The Council set up a Smart House in September 2000 which was equipped with a range of different technologies including more advanced social alarm technology, lifestyle monitoring devices, social/communication technology, Telemedicine (medical monitoring) equipment and environmental control equipment.

The Smart House itself was a self-contained, fully furnished and wheelchair-accessible, two-bedroom bungalow which in former times had been a warden's house attached to Sheltered Housing. The latter had then later been converted into the project's pilot Housing with Care complex. There were several purposes for developing a Smart House: to learn more about the infrastructure required for installation, to provide a real location for testing and trialling equipment, to aid the assessment and matching process, to promote awareness and knowledge among staff, clients and their relatives and to promote the West Lothian project both locally and further afield.

Around the same time, it was decided to pilot this enhanced community alarm technology and the aim was to identify 75 people with appropriate needs who could trial a standard 'core package' of equipment (see Table 10.1). These people were to be dispersed householders, and the ownership of the property was immaterial (although permission was required from the landlord before any hardwiring could be undertaken). The vision underpinning this idea was that such a Home Safety and Security Package could potentially be of benefit to anyone living in the community, irrespective of age, need or disability, and it was important to test this out.

Home care technologies can provide a spectrum of services to an individual within their own home, and independence may be supported in a number of different ways, including introducing a specialist piece of equipment, alterations to the existing environment and modifying existing equipment. Technology at home may perform different functions such as client safety (risk management), client support and assistance, emergency monitoring and response and client screening and assessment (Williams, 2002a, b). These areas will now be discussed in more detail.

Client safety

Concerns over a person's safety at home are often paramount, and it is often necessary to find ways to manage or reduce risks to the individual as they go about their daily life at home. Technology can act as a safety net allowing the person to continue activities which would otherwise be considered unsafe.

Client support and assistance

Technology can promote continued independence for people who are affected by a whole range of physical or mental health problems. It can also promote the learning of new skills, increase social interactions/networks and sometimes also assist the person to regain lost abilities/roles.

Emergency monitoring and response

The capacity for the automatic detection of emergency situations can relieve anxieties about personal or environmental accidents at home while also necessitating the pre-planning of response arrangements.

Client screening and assessment

Functional assessments typically comprise observation and discussion with involved parties, but cannot give the 24-hour picture, which makes it difficult to assess accurately the degree of risk or trace daily patterns of behaviour. There is future potential for lifestyle monitoring equipment to inform the assessment in a more detailed, comprehensive and therefore more accurate way as this technology can give discrete, longitudinal data which can also inform if someone deviates from normal behaviour patterns, for example in the event of an infection.

The project used a home unit which had the ability to be flexibly programmed for both active and passive use and which could therefore be tailored to suit each individual's situation. It was compatible with a range of peripheral devices which provided personal or environmental protection, for example flood and heat detectors, radio pull cord in a bathroom or a wandering alarm or fall detector. Calls for help could be routed via a control centre or more unusually to a carer nearby (useful in the case of people who wander or who are liable to incontinence, for example), with the system automatically then diverting to the control centre if there were no reply from the carer. When a problem was detected, the control centre's information system told the operator exactly which trigger had raised each call so they instantly knew which detector had been activated and its location before they attempted to make speech contact with the person. The control centre then employed its specifically agreed protocols for intervention – they could call a local key-holder to respond or contact the emergency services depending on the type of call raised. The home unit could be programmed to meet specific needs. It had an intruder alarm facility, could be used as a hands-free telephone with one-touch dialling, remote answering, voice prompts and caller display and therefore the user had the opportunity to be as involved with the technology as they wished, or were able, to be. In the case of a person with dementia, for example, who may be unable to actively operate/engage in the process, the technology would still provide protection, by monitoring the situation and alerting help accordingly.

Recruitment of clients

To further the development of the project, a specialist Home Support Team was appointed in April 2001. The team was led by the policy and development officer and project manager for the Opening Doors Project. An occupational therapist seconded to the team was responsible for helping social work practitioners and community occupational therapists identify any potential need for technology. The remit called for an enthusiastic, flexible and educational approach, much of the early work being to 'spread the word' and encourage practitioners to try using the Home Support Team to pilot technological solutions. They were encouraged to make contact to discuss situational problems, risks or concerns with the occupational therapist, who would provide advice on the most appropriate way forward – whether to run with a traditional solution or to try the new approach. A joint visit would then take place with the referring practitioner to meet the client and further discuss the issues. It was necessary to explain to clients the experimental nature of the work and to establish their willingness to be involved in the pilot project.

The client was advised that much of the technology was developmental in nature and therefore they would be assisting the partners in the project by their participation and willingness to contribute by giving feedback. They were advised that the provision of any technology would be free of charge for the duration of the project but that there would likely be a charge for the service at some time in the future.

Assessment process

In conjunction with the client, the client's family and the referring practitioner, the occupational therapist identified the priorities for attention and the main aims of intervention. A specialist technical assessment was devised, noting the above and the rationale for suggested solutions. It was necessary to take into consideration issues such as life choices, routines and patterns of living, support networks and personal preferences. Also it was essential to examine the physical environment, for example location of sockets, types of door locks and the geography of the house. A report was then compiled with initial thoughts and recommendations and sent to the project manager.

The next stage in the process was a further visit to the client with a technical consultant in attendance. The occupational therapist was responsible for briefing the consultant on the relevant issues and previous discussions and for ensuring that the client was as fully involved in the process as possible. The technical consultant then made recommendations for technical solutions according to needs identified during assessment. These final recommendations were then passed to the project manager for authorisation.

Implementing recommendations

Once authorisation was given, the equipment was ordered and the papers passed to one of four Home Support Team workers. These staff performed a keyworker role, supporting clients prior to, during and post-installation. This involved regular visits and contacts with the client, giving further information, explanations or reassurance, completing relevant documentation and generally providing an ongoing supportive and educative role. The aim was also that these support workers would fulfil a more generic role with the focus on capacity building and being a 'link in the chain of care'. Members of the team were crucial, too, for providing feedback to the management group as the process developed and each had a major responsibility for portraying an enthusiasm about the potential benefits to clients and their families. When interviewed for research purposes, staff reported that they found the most enjoyable part of their work was in spending time with clients and that the feeling they could make a difference to their lives was important. There was also reported to be a general excitement and 'buzz' about being involved in the project, especially as West Lothian was seen as leading the way in the field (Bowes and McColgan, 2001).

The matching process: identifying need

An analysis of the home environment is a necessary part of the individual's unique assessment, and Hagedorn (2000) details an approach to this core concern of occupational therapists in the chapter on environmental analysis and adaptation. Specific medical conditions may lead to specific risks and disabilities can increase the risk of accidents in the home (Hagedorn, 2000). For example, poor mobility increases the risk of falls and therefore the potential for lying undetected on the floor for some hours. In the case of dementia, this condition increases the chances of someone leaving the cooker on with a pan burning dry, forgetting about a lit cigarette or the possibility that they go wandering outdoors during the night inappropriately dressed. As people stay longer in the community, there are new roles for occupational therapists and frontline care staff as they try to manage these situations. This requires imagination and lateral thinking to problem solve. In other words, it necessitates searching for original or inspirational ways to find solutions to problems, either by traditional means or using newer methods of matching technology to needs (Astrid, 2000). There is a need to identify risk reduction techniques, be this by teaching, action or other intervention.

Despite the fact that there may be a similarity of diagnosis, it is vital that every person is treated as a unique individual. There is no common prescription for similar situations, because every assessment has a unique client at its centre. It is important to identify needs rather than to simply focus on diagnosis or eligibility for services. The skill in assessment for technology is in thinking around every application and anticipating the pitfalls before they arise. For example, a fall detector may be quickly assumed to be the solution for someone with a history of falling, but it has to be considered manageable for the person to wear or its use needs to be supported by the person's package of care. Using the same example, routines and individual rhythms of life need to be explored since a fall detector may be contraindicated if the person routinely falls asleep lying down on the bed or sofa during the day. Likewise, a wandering alarm may seem the ideal solution to reduce a proven risk but if there is nobody locally to respond immediately by guiding the person home it may not be an appropriate solution.

Case study 10.1

Usage of technology also involves the unpredictable human element. A real situation arose early on when an elderly couple were provided with technology as part of the pilot project. He was frail and extremely deaf; she had advanced dementia. There were numerous potential risks identified for this couple including the possibility of fires from a cigarette lighter, intruders due to an unlocked front door, he had a history of falls and she had demonstrated an inability to call for help if her husband required assistance, even with him shouting instructions. By the time she had reached the phone and dialled a number, she had forgotten why she was using the phone. It was agreed to pilot some technology with this couple and the core package plus some extras were installed.

The woman was having a wash in the bathroom. She dropped the soap, bent to pick it up and carried on washing herself. Her husband meantime was struggling to hear the control centre operator, who was attempting to ask him if there was a flood in the bathroom. It transpired that the flood detector was bobbing around in the basin of water and the soap was still on the floor!

In this case, the couple moved on to long-term care not long after technology was provided. We learned from this that earlier provision is desirable to allow people the opportunity to become familiar with and understand the equipment before it is an emergency need. Although the technology did serve to give them additional protection for a time, the benefits would have been greater had it been available to them much earlier.

Case study 10.2
Technology has also been invaluable in some unexpected situations. A call was received from a man who was praising the fact that he had recently been provided with a Home Safety package of equipment. He was wearing his pendant and the personal trigger button was pressed. The control centre were connected but were unable to hear any verbal response from him.

The nearest key-holder was called and on arrival was searching without success for the man, who, it transpired, had been trapped in his garden shed when the door had slammed shut behind him.

Case study 10.3
On another occasion, a woman who had also had a Home Safety package installed was contacted by the control centre when her flood detector raised the alarm. It emerged that she had been defrosting her freezer, had slipped on the wet floor and was lying fallen in the kitchen. She had been unable to reach her personal trigger but the flood detector raising an alarm call resulted in her being able to receive assistance from a key-holder to get up from the floor.

Case study 10.4
A very independent 91-year-old woman had been experiencing numerous crashing falls at home which had usually resulted in her needing medical attention. She was becoming very upset that her position at home was becoming tenuous. She was provided with a core package of Home Safety equipment and a fall detector to wear around her waist.

For the following two years, she has had no further falls. Although the precise reason for this is unclear, the current hypothesis is that she has gained in confidence and this has resulted in improved posture and gait. She continues to live independently in her own home and says that 'the technology is out of this world and the staff are marvellous'.

When considering whether or not it is appropriate to use technology as part of the care package, Bjornaby et al. (1999) identify nine steps in the decision-making process. At the outset, it was found that these principles provided a helpful baseline for trialling technology, and staff still continue to find the framework helpful in rolling out the now mainstream Home Safety Service.

Living circumstances

When assessing anyone for technology (or any other service), a holistic approach to assessment is required. A full picture needs to be assimilated on the person's domestic situation. The more information that can be gleaned about their health, affects of any disability on their lifestyle, risks/challenges experienced and environmental constraints, the better.

Individual needs of the person

The aim would be to establish needs using a person-centred approach, looking to identify both the things that are difficult and the things that the person would like to be able to manage. Carers will have views too on the situation.

Identify the problems

What are the risks to the person? (See also Chapter 8.) There is a need to clarify whether reported episodes are isolated incidents or recurrent in nature. Isolated incidents usually require no action. The situation could be having a negative impact on the person but again, if not, there may be no need to do anything. Here a conflict of interest may be observed between what the person views as a risk/problem and how their carer perceives the situation.

Identify appropriate goals/interventions

Plan with the person the best way forward, establishing co-operation and consent and always giving due consideration to low-tech and traditional solutions first. Intervention should be flexible and uniquely tailored to the needs of the individual. The potential benefits to carers may also need to be considered at this point.

Ethical dilemmas

It is useful to identify whether technology is more or less ethical than any other solution, for example locking someone into their home or using cot sides to act as restraints. Consideration should be given to the motives involved and the implications of any intervention on privacy and intrusion. Bjornaby et al. (1999, p. 13) suggest that the following questions should help inform ethical decision-making:

(i) Can it be morally acceptable to make safety-increasing alterations in the home of a person with dementia against their wishes because it is believed this would make them better off?

(ii) Is it acceptable if there is a potential danger to self or others?

(iii) May carers deceive a person with dementia to increase his/her safety and well-being?

(iv) Is it more acceptable to leave known risks unaddressed or to employ means of restraint or monitoring?

(v) As with any OT intervention, informed consent is required to install monitoring equipment (COT, 2005) so under what circumstances could it seem acceptable to use this method of risk management?

In recording these dilemmas the legal/professional guidance over client records applies.

Assess and recommend technology

When formulating ideas about services and creating a plan for action, it is necessary to consider the person's right to self-determination, the right to fair treatment/intervention versus duty of care and the person's right to refuse input and to receive respect for making such a decision.

Choose and decide on solutions

As part of the process of gaining informed consent, the client will require information on how the equipment works or any implications of its application as well as any identified pros/cons of the chosen solutions (COT, 2005).

Implementation

Think about the implications of installation, time, disruption involved etc., the need for support, teaching, troubleshooting and the responsibility for servicing and maintenance. Consider duties under Provision and Use of Work Equipment Regulations (HSE, 1999), as technology always has the potential to go wrong. It may be desirable for the funding authority to devise legal documents outlining terms of provision and installation, particularly if the building's infrastructure will be affected.

Evaluation

As in any occupational therapy treatment plan it is essential to revisit the initial aims to see whether the identified needs have been adequately met and then to modify them as appropriate and build in a mechanism for ongoing support and evaluation. It has proved highly beneficial and supportive to have an infrastructure which includes a dedicated team of staff and to use a keyworker system in order to effectively process the review and modification of the intervention.

The matching process: matching technology to needs identified

The range of service users who may benefit from technology at home means that often people have very complex support needs. They should have access to assessment of the highest quality. Research has demonstrated that technology can be effective for a range of particularly challenging circumstances (Bowes and McColgan, 2003).

At the outset of the Opening Doors Project, it seemed to be difficult to identify possible service users who should receive potential benefit from technology. It is thought that the reason for this was partly due to difficulties experienced by mainstream assessment staff in grasping the new concept and in understanding how technology could be used to good effect with people having complex needs. Following the aforementioned training, referrals to the project were more forthcoming and the author routinely encouraged joint assessment visits with referring agents to aid understanding and promote discussion and enthusiasm for the idea.

Technology assessments are not carried out in isolation but rather form a specialist part of the Community Care Assessment process. In the future there will clearly be a need to link any such technology assessment to a single shared assessment process. The use of assistive/supportive technologies should not be seen as something separate from normal provision but rather as an addition to the range of supportive options which are currently available. The aim of this approach may make technology more acceptable and familiar to assessment staff and minimise possible 'cultural' resistance to technology in principle.

There is no common recipe for provision, because every assessment has a unique individual at its core. In other words, two clients with the same diagnosis may be assessed as having quite different needs and, while a core package of Home Safety equipment is recognised to have benefit to all irrespective of age or disability, the personal prescription added onto this core package would in all probability be totally different and entirely dependent on each individual's situation, interests and support needs. Focusing on the specific needs of the individual and not adopting a 'one size fits all' approach is important.

As with any assessment, decisions must be made in consultation with the client and the main priorities for intervention established. It would not be desirable to swamp the person with too much technology, far better to start small and add to the prescription as familiarity/needs/ enthusiasm develops. Technology should be viewed as an addition to existing services and support structures, not as a replacement for these. The assessment must take into consideration many of the human factors and operating or budgetary constraints that will influence the final choice of care technologies provided.

Evaluation and review

Following the installation of technology, there needs to be ongoing support and evaluation of its sustainability or otherwise. Invariably, there are anxieties at the start, which makes it necessary to support people with its introduction into their home environment. Depending on the types of technology prescribed and the interest and ability of the user to be involved in its usage, repeat demonstrations and skill/interest development will be a large part of the support team's remit. In the event of fault or breakdown, reassurance and practical assistance will be required. Good record-keeping tracking past and present interventions is essential. The use of an individual care plan including goal-setting and the identification of longer-term aims is helpful to keep focused and ensure that the technology is still appropriate and meeting the initial needs.

The wide-scale application of technological in the community setting requires a responsive and efficient repairs process. Since individuals' safety depends on equipment working reliably, it has to be functioning at optimal levels and there has to be a contingency in the event of any piece of equipment becoming dysfunctional. Servicing and maintenance agreements need to be established by managers with clinical experience to incorporate cleaning of equipment such as smoke sensors, annual battery replacements and upgrade/replacement of equipment as and when appropriate. The charging policy may need to be reviewed at a later date to sustain the service. After seven years, it is planned that key components will be upgraded. Technological development moves on apace. Since the start of the project, devices have moved from being hardwired to radio-based wireless technology (making installation easier, cheaper and less intrusive). Recently, too, the radio frequency has changed resulting in the need for an upgraded home unit and another range of frequency-compatible sensors. An imminent future upgrade to the home unit will offer new functionality including a medication reminder facility and the ability to create zoned areas for intruder detection.

In evaluation, it has become apparent that there are clear benefits for clients and their carers. In research, the overwhelmingly consistent viewpoint was that the technology gave additional peace of mind.

It is not solely about staying at home but helping people recognise their strengths rather than focusing on what they cannot do. It has been found that this type of assistance enables carers to care for longer, with the result that the person is able to live at home for longer. In West Lothian, the duration of stay in nursing homes has reduced from an average of 3.2 years to 1.3 years since the project began. The use of technology in the home environment has been influential in this change in trend, as have better availability of community rehabilitation and the development of enhanced home care services. Technology has provided reassurance for clients and has promoted independence allowing tasks previously viewed as dangerous to the individual to be carried out with reduced risk. The use of technology has helped to postpone what might otherwise have been an inevitable move elsewhere and has given clients another choice. The home environment has been made safer for clients and the stress has been reduced for carers. It has made a holistic improvement to the quality of someone's life rather than just service provision (Bowes and McColgan, 2003).

Current developments in smart housing

One of the things learned from the pilot project is that the earlier technology is introduced, the better, in order that people have the opportunity to become accustomed to having it in their homes while it is an asset to overall protection rather than an assessed need. We are now offering the Home Safety Service to all people over the age of 60 who wish to have the technology installed in their home. The service is marketed as a safety and security system, without an emphasis on personal needs. The vision is that, as people become older and more frail and as specific needs develop, the core technology can be enhanced through the addition of specific devices to address assessed needs.

Currently, an electronic standardised assessment tool is being devised for specialist technology assessment in conjunction with single shared assessment. The development of a risk and safety assessment capable of identifying appropriate assistive and telecare technologies/services is complex. It will be necessary to consider aspects relating to the client, the home generally, the specific rooms in use, tasks undertaken and behaviours, then to identify key assessment parameters and scores to implement aspects of the risk assessment procedure following overview assessment. A pilot of the prototype software will be used to obtain initial user feedback from potential assessors and clients in West Lothian in order to ensure that the tool is suited to the needs of frontline assessors. It will be piloted using a tablet PC with a planned timescale of several months' duration.

Assuming a successful pilot, the standardised assessment will be marketed as a tool for the assessment of both care needs and, more specifically, technology needs with the aim of promoting greater accuracy of assessment and ultimately enable home living for longer, in greater safety and with maximum independence.

Good communication continues to be important with ongoing close communication between technicians, clinicians and care staff. Only by our specifying to the technicians what is required to address complex needs can they work on developing new ways to manage problem areas. Technicians then depend on clinicians and clients to test out new products for reliability and effectiveness. This two-way process of communication aids the introduction of newly marketed products, for example there will shortly be a field trial of a bed sensor for people with epilepsy, which creates an alert via the home unit.

It is important to make both the general public and frontline council staff aware of the potential benefits of technology to ensure that everyone who is eligible and who wishes to can apply for the service. This is done by featuring the Home Safety Service in a range of publications/flyers, generating media coverage and holding roadshows/workshops giving presentations and demonstrations of the technology in action.

Key points

- Technology in its different forms can be used with a whole spectrum of client groups adding another dimension to independent living. The application of technology requires occupational therapy assessment and intervention approaches, as outlined elsewhere in the text. It is simply another tool for enabling people to live independently.
- The use of assistive/supportive technologies should not be seen as something separate from normal provision but rather as an addition to the range of supportive options which are currently available.
- It has occupational benefits, for example education or productivity and earning a living, self-care or managing life or leisure/pleasure activities, and contributes to the work–life balance.
- Technology offers new solutions to occupational disruptions and may reduce the need for dependence on others for personal and domestic activities of daily living.
- As people stay longer in the community, there are new roles for therapists and frontline care staff as they try and manage these situations.

This often requires imagination and lateral thinking to problem-solve. In other words, it necessitates searching for original or inspirational ways to find solutions to problems, either by traditional means or using newer methods of matching technology to needs.

* Despite the fact that there may be a similarity of diagnosis, it is vital that every person is treated as a unique individual. There is no common recipe for provision, because every assessment has a unique individual at its core. Focusing on the specific needs of the individual and not adopting a 'one size fits all' approach is important.

* Technology is not always the answer, and good assessment is the key to identifying needs which can genuinely be matched to helpful technology. For example, a sensor to detect wandering behaviour may be quickly assumed to be the solution for someone with a history of wandering. However, if there is nobody in the immediate vicinity who is available to respond by going out to find the person, there is an immediate problem and installing a wandering sensor may not be the best way to manage the situation.

* The appropriate use of technology helps to provide a safety net, reducing the threat to the person of being removed into care at an early stage.

* The technology gives additional peace of mind to clients and their carers. It is not solely about staying at home but helping people recognise and maintain their strengths as opposed to focusing on what they cannot do. It allows people to perform necessary/therapeutic tasks in a safer way.

References

Abberley P (1993) Disabled people and 'normality'. In J Swain, V Finkelstein, S French et al. (eds), Disabling Barriers – Enabling Environments. Milton Keynes: Sage.

Abberley P (1995) Disabling ideology in health and welfare – the case of occupational therapy. Disability and Society 10(2): 221–32.

Abberley P (2004) A critique of professional support and intervention. In J Swain, S French, C Barnes et al. (eds), Disabling Barriers – Enabling Environments (2nd edn.). London: Sage.

Abraham B, Clamp S (1991) Aids and adaptations: a new practice model, Part 1. British Journal of Occupational Therapy 54(9): 341–5.

Adams J (1996) Adapting for community care, Part 2. British Journal of Occupational Therapy 59(4): 185–7.

Allen C, Milner J, Price D (2002) Home is Where the Start Is: The housing and Urban Experiences of Visually Impaired Children. York: Joseph Rowntree Foundation.

ASA A117.1 (1961) American Standard Specifications for Making Buildings and Facilities Accessible to and Usable by the Physically Handicapped. New York: American Standards Association.

Astrid (2000) ASTRID: introducing assistive technology. A social and technological response to meeting the needs of individuals with dementia. Journal of Dementia Care 8(4): 18–19.

Atkinson N, Crawforth M (1995) All in the Family: Siblings and Disability. London: NCH Action for Children.

Audit Commission (1998) Home Alone: The Role of Housing and Community Care. London: The Audit Commission.

Awang D (2002) Older people and participation within disabled facilities grant processes. British Journal of Occupational Therapy 65(6): 261–8.

Awang D (2004) Building in Evidence: Reviewing Housing and Occupational Therapy. London: College of Occupational Therapists.

BackCare (1999) Safer Handling of People in the Community. Teddington: National Back Pain Association.

Baldock J, Manning N, Miller S et al. (1999) Social Policy. Oxford: Oxford University Press.

Barnes C (1991) Disabled People in Britain and Discrimination: A Case for Anti-discrimination Legislation. London: Hurst.

Barnes C, Mercer G (eds) (1997) Doing Disability Research. Leeds: The Disability Press.

Barnes C, Mercer G (2003) Disability. Cambridge: Polity Press.

Barnes C, Mercer G, Shakespeare T (1999) Exploring Disability: A Sociological Introduction. Cambridge: Polity Press.

Beresford B, Oldman C (2002) Housing Matters: National Evidence Relating to Disabled Children and Their Housing. Bristol: Policy Press.

Best R (1997) The housing dimension. In M Benzeval, K Judge, M Whitehead (eds), Tackling Inequalities in Health: An Agenda for Action. London: The King's Fund.

Bevan M (2002) Housing and Disabled Children: The Art of the Possible. Bristol: Policy Press.

Bjornaby S, Topo P, Holthe T (1999) Technology, Ethics and Dementia – A Guidebook on How to Apply Technology in Dementia Care. Oslo, Norway: The Norwegian Centre for Dementia Research.

Blythe A, O'Brien P, McDaid S (2002) Lifetime Homes in Northern Ireland: Evolution or Revolution. Belfast: Joseph Rowntree Foundation/Chartered Institute of Housing (NI).

Bowes A, McColgan G (2001) Evaluation of Opening Doors for Older People in West Lothian. University of Stirling.

Bowes A, McColgan G (2003) Opening Doors for Older People: Evaluation of Programmes for Housing With Care in 'Wired' West Lothian. Interim Report. Department of Applied Social Science, University of Stirling.

Bowes A, McColgan G (2005) Smart Technology at Home: Users' and Carers' Perspectives. Interim Report – February 2005. West Lothian Council and the University of Stirling.

Bowling A (1997) Measuring Health: A Review of Quality of Life Measurement Scales. 2nd edn. Buckingham: Open University Press.

Bowling A (2001) Measuring Disease (2nd edn.). Buckingham: Open University Press.

Brewerton J, Darton D (1997) Designing Lifetime Homes. York: Joseph Rowntree Foundation.

Briggs L (1993) Striving for Independence. In J Swain, V Finkelstein, S French et al. (eds), Disabling Barriers – Enabling Environments. London: Sage.

British Standards Institution (2001) BS: 8300 Design of Buildings and Their Approaches to Meet the Needs of Disabled People – Code of Practice. Milton Keynes: British Standards Institution.

Buckle P, Randle PM (1989) An Ergonomic Model. University of Surrey. <www.eihms.surrey.ac.uk/robens/erg/inclusivedesignmodule/module9/intro.pdf>, accessed 15/12/04.

Bull R (1998a) Housing Options for Disabled People. London: Jessica Kingsley Publishers.

Bull R (1998b) Making the most of an occupational therapist's skills in housing for people with disabilities. In R Bull (ed.), Housing Options for Disabled People. London: Jessica Kingsley Publishers.

Burns N (2000) Access all tenures: barriers to home ownership for disabled people. Housing in the 21st Century: Fragmentation or Reorientation? International Conference. Sweden: Gavle.

Bury T, Mead J (1998) Evidence Based Healthcare. Oxford: Butterworth-Heinemann.

Calnan S, Sixma HJ, Calnan MW et al. (2000) Quality of local authority occupational therapy services: developing an instrument to measure the user's perspective. British Journal of Occupational Therapy 63(4): 155–62.

CAOT (Canadian Association of Occupational Therapists) (1997) Enabling Occupations: An Occupational Therapy Perspective. Ottawa: CAOT Publications.

Carroll C, Cowans J, Darton D (1999) Meeting Part M and Designing Lifetime Homes. York: Joseph Rowntree Foundation.

Chapparo C, Ranka J (2000) Clinical reasoning in occupational therapy. In J Higgs, M Jones (2000) Clinical Reasoning in the Health Professions (2nd edn.). Oxford: Butterworth-Heinemann.

Chard G (2004) International classification of functioning, disability and health. British Journal of Occupational Therapy 67(1): 1.

Christiansen CH, Baum CM (1997) Occupational Therapy: Enabling Function and Well Being (2nd edn.). Thorofare, NJ: Slack.

CIPFA (1996) Benchmarking to Improve Performance. London: Chartered Institute of Public Finance and Accountancy.

Clemson L (1997) Home Fall Hazards and the Westmead Home Safety Assessment. West Brunswick, Australia: Coordinates Publications. 6.

Clements L, Read J (2003) Disabled People and European Human Rights. Bristol: Policy Press.

Clemson L, Roland M, Cumming R (1992) Occupational therapy assessment of potential hazards in the homes of elderly people: an inter-relater reliability study. Australian Occupational Therapy Journal 39(3): 23–6.

Clemson L, Fitzgerald M, Heard R (1999) Content validity of an assessment tool to identify home fall hazards: The Westmead Home Safety Assessment. British Journal of Occupational Therapy 62(4): 171–9.

Cobbold C (1997) A Cost Benefit Analysis of Lifetime Homes. York: Joseph Rowntree Foundation.

COT (College of Occupational Therapists) (2001a) Outcome Measures: Information Pack for Occupational Therapy. London: COT.

COT (College of Occupational Therapists) (2001b) Code of Ethics and Professional Conduct for Occupational Therapists. British Journal of Occupational Therapy 64(12): 612–17.

COT (College of Occupational Therapists) (2002) From Interface to Integration. A Strategy for Modernising Occupational Therapy Services in Local Health and Social Care Communities. London: COT.

COT (College of Occupational Therapists) (2005) Code of Ethics and Professional Conduct. London: COT.

COTSSIH (College of Occupational Therapists Specialist Section in Housing) (2003) Conference. Access Matters New Directives, Changing Roles. 20–21 October 2003. London: COTSSIH.

COTSSIH (College of Occupational Therapists Specialist Section in Housing) (2004) Research and Development Strategic Vision and Action Plan. London: COT.

Corcoran C, Gitlin L (1997) The role of the physical environment in occupational performance. In CH Christiansen, CM Baum (eds), Occupational Therapy: Enabling Function and Wellbeing. Thorofare, NJ: Slack.

Corlett EN, McAtamney L (1992) Making an Ergonomic Workplace Assessment in a Health Care Context. Institute of Occupational Ergonomics, University of Nottingham.

CABO/ANSI (Council of American Building Officials, and American National Standards Institute) (1992) A117.1-1992 American National Standard: Accessible and Usable Buildings and Facilities. New York: ANSI.

Council of Europe (1950) The European Convention on Human Rights. Rome. <http://www.hri.org/docs/ECHR50.html>, accessed 24/04/03.

Craddock J (1996a) Responses of the occupational therapy profession to the perspective of the disability movement, Part 1. British Journal of Occupational Therapy 59(1): 17–22.

Craddock J (1996b) Responses of the occupational therapy profession to the perspective of the disability movement, Part 2. British Journal of Occupational Therapy 59(2): 73–9.

Creek J (2003) Occupational Therapy Defined as a Complex Intervention. London: COT.

Davis K (1981) 28–38 Grove Road: accommodation and care in a community setting. In A Brechin, P Liddiard, J Swain (eds), Handicap in a Social World. London: Hodder & Stoughton.

Davis K (1993) The crafting of good clients. In J Swain, V Finkelstein, S French et al. (eds), Disabling Barriers – Enabling Environments. Milton Keynes: Sage.

Dean H, Taylor-Gooby P (1992) Dependency Culture: The Explosion of a Myth. London: Harvester Wheatsheaf.

DoE (Department of the Environment) (1974) HDD Occasional Paper 2/74 Mobility Housing Part 8. London: TSO.

DoE (Department of the Environment), Transport and the Regions (1999) The Building Regulations 1991. (1999 edition) Approved document M: Access and Facilities for Disabled People. London: TSO.

DoH (Department of Health) (1997) The New NHS. Modern, Dependable. London: TSO.

DoH (Department of Health) (1998) Modernising Social Services. London: TSO.

DoH (Department of Health) (1998) Quality first. London: DoH.

DoH (Department of Health) (2000a) The NHS Plan 2000: A plan for investment. A plan for reform. Cm 4818-1. London: DoH.

DoH (Department of Health) (2000b) The NHS Plan: The Government's response to the Royal Commission on Long Term Care. <www.dh.gov.uk/PublicationsAnd Statistics/Publications/PublicationsPolicyAndGuidance/PublicationsPolicyAndGui danceArticle/fs/en?CONTENT_ID=4002674&chk=8MsfL0>, accessed 06/04/05.

DoH (Department of Health) (2001) Fair Access to Care Services – Background and Process. <www.dh.gov.uk>, accessed 31/03/05.

DoH (Department of Health) (2002a) Fair Access to Care Services. Guidance on Eligibility Criteria for Adult Social Care. London: Department of Health.

DoH (Department of Health) (2002b) National Service Framework for Older People. London: Department of Health.

DoH/DSS (Department of Health and Department of Social Security) (1989) Caring for People – Community Care in the Next Decade and Beyond 1989. London: TSO.

DoH/SSI (Department of Health and Social Services Inspectorate) (1991) Care Management and Assessment: Practitioners' Guide. London: TSO.

Department of Health, Social Services and Public Safety/Northern Ireland Housing Executive (2002) Joint Fundamental Review of the Housing Adaptations Service. Belfast: Northern Ireland Housing Executive.

DTI (Department of Trade and Industry) (2001) Working for a Safer World: 23rd Annual Report of the Home and Leisure Accident Surveillance System. London: Department of Trade and Industry.

Dewsbury G, Clarke K, Hughes J et al. (2003) Growing Older Digitally: Designing Technology for Older People. Departments of Computing and Sociology, Lancaster University.

Dimond B (1997) Legal Aspects of Occupational Therapy. Oxford: Blackwell Science.

DLF Hamilton Index (latest 2003) Access to Indoor and Outdoor Environments, Part 2 Section 10. Disabled Living Foundation.

Dodd T (1998) Regulations, standards, design guides and plans. In R Bull (ed.), Housing Options for Disabled People. London: Jessica Kingsley Publishers.

Doyal L, Gough I (1991) A Theory of Human Need. Basingstoke: Macmillan.

Drake RF (1996) Understanding Disability Policies. Basingstoke: Macmillan.

Dreyfuss H (1959) The Measure of Man: Human Factors in Design. New York: Whitney Library of Design.

Eakin P, Baird H (1995) The Community Dependency Index: a standardised assessment of need and measure of outcome for community occupational therapy. British Journal of Occupational Therapy 58(1): 17–22.

Esmond D, Gordon K, McCaskie C et al. (1998) More Scope for Fair Housing. London: Scope.

Evans J (2003) The Independent Living Movement in the UK. Independent Living Institute. <www.independentliving.org/docs6/evans2003.html>, accessed 18/02/05.

Finkelstein V (1993) Disability: a social challenge or an administrative responsibility? In J Swain, V Finkelstein, S French et al. (eds), Disabling Barriers – Enabling Environments. Milton Keynes: Sage.

Finlay B (1978) Housing and Disability: A Report on the Housing Needs of Physically Handicapped People in Rochdale. Rochdale Voluntary Action.

Fleming M (1991) The therapist with the 3-track mind. American Journal of Occupational Therapy 45(11): 1007–14.

Fortune T, Ryan S (1996) Applying clinical reasoning: a caseload management system for community occupational therapists. British Journal of Occupational Therapists 59(5): 207–11.

Franklin BJ (1998) Forms and functions: assessing housing need in the community care context. Health and Social Care in the Community 6(6): 420–8.

Frazer R, Glick G (2001) Out of Services: A Survey of Social Service Provision for Elderly and Disabled People in England. London: RADAR.

French S (1994) Attitudes of health professionals towards disabled people: a discussion and review of the literature. Physiotherapy 80(10): 697–93.

French S, Gillman M, Swain J (1997) Working with Visually Disabled People: Bridging Theory and Practice. Birmingham: Venture Press.

Gans H (1968) People and Plans: Essays on Urban Problems and Solutions. New York: Basic Books.

Gibbs K, Barnitt R (1999) Occupational therapy and the self-care needs of Hindu elders. British Journal of Occupational Therapy 62(3): 100–5.

Goldsmith S (1974) Housing Development Directorate Occasional Paper 2/74.

Goldsmith S (1963) Designing for the Disabled. London: RIBA (rev. 1967, 1976, 1984).

Goldsmith S (1997) Designing for the Disabled: The New Paradigm. Oxford: Butterworth-Heinemann.

Goldsmith S (2001) The Bottom Up Methodology of Universal Design. In W Preiser, E Ostroff (2001) Universal Design Handbook. New York: McGraw-Hill.

Goldsmith S, Morton J (1975) Housing Development Directorate Occasional Paper 2/75 Wheelchair Housing (reprinted from the Architects' Journal, 25 June 1975). London: DoE.

Goodridge C (2004) Housing: A Contemporary View of Disabled People's Experience, Provision and Policy Directions. Disability Rights Commission Housing Report. Mobility Housing (reprinted from the Architects' Journal, 3 July 1974). London: DoE.

Great Britain (1948) National Assistance Act. London: TSO.

Great Britain (1970) Chronically Sick and Disabled Persons Act 1970. London: TSO.

Great Britain (1977) National Health Services Act 1977. London: TSO.

Great Britain (1986) Disabled Persons Act 1986. London: TSO.

Great Britain (1989a) Housing Act 1989. London: TSO.

Great Britain (1989b) Local Government and Housing Act 1989. London: TSO.

Great Britain (1989c) Children Act 1989. London: TSO.

Great Britain (1990) National Health Service and Community Care Act 1990. London: TSO.

Great Britain (1992) Manual Handling Operations Regulations 1992. London: TSO.

Great Britain (1995a) Carers (Recognition and Services) Act 1995. London: TSO.

Great Britain (1995b) The Disability Discrimination Act. London: TSO.

Great Britain (1996a) Housing Grants, Construction and Regeneration Act 1996. London: TSO.

Great Britain (1996b) Community Care (Direct Payments) Act 1996. London: TSO.

Great Britain (1998) Human Rights Act 1998. London: TSO.

Great Britain (1999a) Health Act 1999. London: TSO.

Great Britain (1999b) Local Government Act 1999. London: TSO.

Great Britain (2000) Carers and Disabled Children Act 2000. London: TSO.

Great Britain (2002) Regulatory Reform Order (Housing Assistance) 2002. London: TSO.

Greater London Authority (2004) Accessible London: creating an inclusive environment GLA. <www.london.gov.uk/mayor/strategies/sds/docs/ spg_accessible_london.pdf>, accessed 11/08/04.

Atkinson B, Dodd T (2002) The Greenwich Wheelchair Site Brief. London: Greenwich Housing Disability Team, Greenwich Council.

Habinteg Housing Association (Ulster) Ltd (1996) Design Guide Appendices. Belfast: Habinteg Housing Association (Ulster).

Habinteg Housing Association (2005) Design Guides. Habinteg Housing Association. <www.habinteg.org.uk/pages/design_guides.html>, accessed 01/03/05.

Hagedorn R (1995) Occupational Therapy: Perspectives and Processes. Edinburgh: Churchill Livingstone.

Hagedorn R (2000) Tools for Practice in Occupational Therapy: A Structured Approach to Core Skills and Processes. Edinburgh: Churchill Livingstone.

Hagedorn R (2001) Occupational Therapy: Foundations for Practice (3rd edn.). Edinburgh: Churchill Livingstone.

Harrison M (2003) From Gans to Coleman to the social model of disability: physical environmental determinism revisited. Paper given at Seminar for The Social Model of Disability: health and social support services. Weetwood Hall, Leeds, 17 September.

Hasselkus B (2002) The Meaning of Everyday Occupation. Thorofare, NJ: Slack.

Hawker M, King N (1999) An Ordinary Home: Housing and Support for People with Learning Disabilities. London: IDEA Publications.

Hawkins R, Stewart S (2002) Changing rooms: the impact of adaptations on the meaning of home for a disabled person and the role of the occupational therapist in the process. British Journal of Occupational Therapy 65(2): 81–7.

HSE (Health and Safety Executive) (1992) Guidance on Manual Handling Regulations. London: HSE.

HSE (Health and Safety Executive) (1999) Provision and Use of Work Equipment Regulations 1998: Open Learning Guidance HSE Books. London: HSE.

Heater D (1990) Citizenship: the civic ideal in world history, politics and education. Harlow: Longman.

Heaton J, Bamford C (2001) Assessing the outcomes of equipment and adaptations: issues and approaches. British Journal of Occupational Therapy 64(7): 346–56.

Henderson A (1996) The scope of occupational science. In R Zemke, F Clarke (1996) Occupational Science: The Evolving Discipline. Philadelphia: FA Davis.

Hèrbert M, Thibeault R, Landry A et al. (2000) Introducing an evaluation of community based occupational therapy services: a client-centred practice. Canadian Journal of Occupational Therapy 67(3): 146–54.

Heywood F (1994) Adaptations: Finding Ways to Say Yes. Bristol: SAUS Publications.

Heywood F (2001) Money Well Spent: The Effectiveness and Value of Housing Adaptations. Bristol: Policy Press.

Heywood F (2004) The health outcomes of housing adaptations. Disability and Society 19(2):129–43.

Higgs J, Jones M (2000) Clinical Reasoning in the Health Professions (2nd edn.). Oxford: Butterworth-Heinemann.

Hogan A (2001) Disability Discrimination: Law and Litigation. Welwyn Garden City: EMS Professional Publishing.

House of Commons Health Committee (2004) Select Committee on Health, Third Report <http://www.parliament.the-stationery-office.co.uk/pa/cm200304/cmselect/cmhealth/23/2302.htm>, accessed 01/08/05.

Hurst R (1990) Independent. In L Laurie (ed.), Building Our Lives: Housing, Independent Living and Disabled People. London: Shelter.

Illich I (1977) Limits to Medicine: medical nemesis, the expropriation of health. New York: Penguin.

Imrie R (1998) Oppression, disability and access in the built environment. In T Shakespeare (ed.), The Disability Reader: Social Science Perspectives. London: Cassell.

Imrie R (2004) From universal to inclusive design in the built environment. In J Swain, S French, C Barnes et al. (eds), Disabling Barriers – Enabling Environments (2nd edn.). London: Sage.

Iwarsson S (1999) The housing enabler: an objective tool for assessing accessibility. British Journal of Occupational Therapy 62(11): 491–7.

Iwarsson S, Fange A, Hovbrandt P et al. (2004) Occupational therapy targeting physical environmental barriers in buildings with public facilities. British Journal of Occupational Therapy 67(1): 29–38.

Jensen J, Mace J, Meghani-Wise Z et al. (1998) Specific areas of work, research or investigation. In R Bull (ed.), Housing Options for Disabled People. London: Jessica Kingsley Publishers.

Johnstone D (1998) An Introduction to Disability Studies. London: David Fulton Publishers.

Jones D, Blair S, Hartery T, et al. (2000) Sociology and Occupational Therapy: An Integrated Approach. Edinburgh: Churchill Livingstone.

Jones LJC (2000) Reshaping welfare: voices from the debate. In C Davies, L Finlay, A Bullman (eds), Changing Practice in Health and Social Care. London: Open University Press/Sage.

Joseph Rowntree Foundation (1998) Assessing Housing Needs in Community Care. York: Joseph Rowntree Foundation.

Judd S (1997) Technology. In M Marshall (ed.), State of the Art in Dementia Care. London: Centre for Policy on Ageing.

Langan M (ed.) (1998) Welfare: Needs, Rights and Risks. London: Routledge/ Open University Press.

Law M, Baptiste S, Carswell A et al. (1994) Canadian Occupational Performance Measure (2nd edn.). Ottawa: CAOT Publications ACE.

Law M, Cooper BA, Strong S et al. (1997) Theoretical contexts for the practice of occupational therapy. In CH Christiansen, CM Baum (eds), Occupational Therapy: Enabling Function and Well Being (2nd edn.). Thorofare, NJ: Slack.

Law M, Baum C, Dunn W (2001) Measuring Occupational Performance: Supporting Best Practice in Occupational Therapy. Thorofare, NJ: Slack.

Leonard P (1997) Postmodern Welfare: Reconstructing an Emancipatory Project. London: Sage.

Letts L, Scott S, Burtney J et al. (1998) The reliability and validity of the Safety Assessment of Function and the Environment for Rehabilitation (SAFER Tool). British Journal of Occupational Therapy 61(3): 127–32.

Liddle J, McKenna K (2000) Quality of life: an overview of issues for use in occupational therapy outcome measurement. Australian Occupational Therapy Journal 47: 77–85.

Lord S, Sherrington C, Menz H (2001) Falls in Older People. Risk Factors and Strategies for Prevention. Cambridge: Cambridge University Press.

Luck R, Haenlein H, Bright K (2001) Project briefing for an inclusive universal design process. In: Preiser W, Ostroff E (eds), Universal Design Handbook. New York: McGraw-Hill.

McCleoud W, Hanks P (eds) (1987) The New Collins Concise English Dictionary. Aylesbury: Bookclub Associates.

McCoy D, Smith M (1992) The Prevalence of Disability among Adults in Northern Ireland. Belfast: Policy Planning and Research Unit, Department of Finance and Personnel.

McDonald R, Surtees R, Wirz S (2004) The international classification of functioning, disability and health provides a model for adaptive seating interventions for children with cerebral palsy. British Journal of Occupational Therapy 67(7): 293–302.

McDowell I, Newell C (1996) Measuring Health: A Guide to Rating Scales and Questionnaires (2nd edn.). Oxford: Oxford University Press.

Macfarlane A, Laurie L (1996) Demolishing 'Special Needs': Fundamental Principles of Non-Discriminatory Housing. Belpar: British Council of Disabled People.

McKeever B (2001) Time to Act: A Family View of Disability. Derry: Family Information Group.

Malin N, Wilmot S, Mabelthorpe J (2002) Key Concepts and Debates in Health and Social Policy. Buckingham: Open University Press.

Mandelstam M (1997) Equipment for Older or Disabled People and the Law. London: Jessica Kingsley Publishers.

Mandelstam M (1998) A question of good practice? Community care law and occupational therapists. British Journal of Occupational Therapy 61(8): 351–8.

Mandelstam M (1999) Community Care Practice and the Law (2nd edn.). London: Jessica Kingsley Publishers.

Marshall M (ed.) (2000) A Social & Technological Response to Meeting the Needs of Individuals with Dementia & Their Carers (ASTRID). London: Hawker Publications.

Martin J, Meltzer H, Elliot D (1988) The Prevalence of Disability Among Adults. London: TSO.

Maslow A (1970) Motivation and Personality (2nd edn.). New York: Harper & Row.

Mattingly C (1991a) What is clinical reasoning? American Journal of Occupational Therapy 45(11): 979–86.

Mattingly C (1991b) The narrative nature of clinical reasoning. American Journal of Occupational Therapy 45(11): 998–1005.

Mattingly C, Gilette N (1991) Anthropology, occupational therapy and action research. American Journal of Occupational Therapy 45(11): 972–8.

Mattingly C, Fleming M (1994) Clinical Reasoning Forms of Inquiry in Therapeutic Practice. Philadelphia: FA Davis.

Medhurst A, Ryan S (1996a) Clinical reasoning in local authority paediatric occupational therapy: planning a major adaptation for the child with a degenerative condition, Part 1. British Journal of Occupational Therapy 59(5):203–6.

Medhurst A, Ryan S (1996b) Clinical reasoning in local authority paediatric occupational therapy: planning a major adaptation for the child with a degenerative condition, Part 2. British Journal of Occupational Therapy 59(6): 269–72.

Meghani-Wise Z (1996) Why this interest in minority ethnic groups? British Journal of Occupational Therapy 59(10): 485–9.

Morris J (1990) Our Homes Our Rights: Housing, Independent Living and Physically Disabled People. London: Shelter.

Morris J (1993) Housing, independent living and physically disabled people. In J Swain, V Finkelstein, S French et al. (eds), Disabling Barriers – Enabling Environments. London: Sage.

Mountain G (2000) Occupational Therapy in Social Services Departments. A Review of the Literature. London: COT.

Mullick A (2001) Universal bathrooms. In W Preiser, E Ostroff (eds), Universal Design Handbook. New York: McGraw-Hill.

Munroe H (1996) Clinical reasoning in community occupational therapy. British Journal of Occupational Therapy 59(5): 196–202.

National Institute for Clinical Excellence (2004) Falls. The Assessment and Prevention of Falls in Older People. Clinical Guideline 21. The National Institute for Clinical Excellence.

NIDDK (National Institute of Diabetes & Digestive & Kidney Diseases) (2004) Publication: Understanding Adult Obesity. <http://win.niddk.nih.gov/publications/understanding.htm>, accessed 11/07/2004.

National Statistics (2005) Ageing: 16% of the UK population are 65 or over. <www.statistics.gov.uk>, accessed 03/03/05.

National Wheelchair Housing Association Group/Home Housing Trust (1997) Wheelchair Housing Design Guide. Watford: Construction Research Communications Ltd.

Neufeldt A (1999) Appearances of disability, discrimination and the transformation of rehabilitation service practices. In R Leavitt (ed.), Cross-cultural Rehabilitation: An International Perspective. London: WB Saunders.

Nirje B (1980) The normalisation principle. In RJ Flynn, KE Nitsch (eds), Normalisation, Social Integration and Community Services. Baltimore: University Park Press.

Nocon A, Pleace N (1997) Until disabled people get consulted: the role of occupational therapy in meeting housing needs. British Journal of Occupational Therapy 60(3): 115–22.

Norman A (1998) Losing your home. In M Allott, M Robb (eds), Understanding Health and Social Care: A Reader. London: Sage.

NIHE (Northern Ireland Housing Executive) (2003a) Inclusive Design through Home Adaptations. A Good Practice Guide. N. Ireland: The Regional Strategic Housing Authority.

NIHE (Northern Ireland Housing Executive) (2003b) Joint Fundamental Review of the Housing Adaptations Service. Belfast: NIHE. Email: maurice. rooney@nihe.gov. uk.

NIHE (Northern Ireland Housing Executive) (2004) Inclusive Design Through Home Adaptations: A Good Practice Guide. Belfast: NIHE.

O'Brien J (1986) A guide to personal futures planning. In GT Bellamy, B Wilcox (eds), The Activities Catalogue: Community Programming for Youth and Adults with Severe Disabilities. Baltimore: Brookes.

O'Brien J (1987) A Guide to lifestyle planning: using the activities catalogue to integrate services and natural support systems. In B Wilcox, GT Bellamy (eds), The Activities Catalogue: An Alternative Curriculum for Youth and Adults with Severe Disabilities. Baltimore: Brookes.

O'Brien P (1999) Perspectives on Whether Housing Design Guidance Recognises the Needs of Disabled People With Severe Mobility Impairments and their Carers. (Unpublished MA Dissertation, COT, Thesis Loan Section).

O'Brien P (2003) Disabled facilities grants: are they meeting the assessed needs of children in Northern Ireland? British Journal of Occupational Therapy 66(6): 277–80.

ODPM (Office of the Deputy Prime Minister) (2004a) Decent Homes – A Tenants Guide. London: ODPM. <www.odpm.gov.uk>, accessed 03/03/05.

ODPM (Office of the Deputy Prime Minister) (2004b) News Release, 13 February 2004: £101m to help disabled people stay in their own home. <www.odpm.gov.uk>, accessed 03/03/05.

ODPM (Office of the Deputy Prime Minister) (2004c) Delivering Housing Adaptations for Disabled People: A Good Practice Guide. London: ODPM, DoH, DES.

ODPM/DoH (Office of the Deputy Prime Minister, Department of Health) (2004) Delivering Adaptations for Disabled People: A Good Practice Guide. London: ODPM.

OHCHR (Office of the High Commissioner for Human Rights) (1948) Universal Declaration of Human Rights. <www.unhchr.ch/udhr/lang/eng.htm>, accessed 24/04/03.

OHCHR (Office of the High Commissioner for Human Rights) (1989) The United Nations Convention on the Rights of the Child 1989. <www.unhchr.ch/html/ menu3/b/ k2crc.htm>, accessed 24/04/03.

Oliver M (1990) The Politics of Disablement. Basingstoke: Macmillan.

Oliver M (1993) Disability and dependency: a creation of industrial societies? In J Swain, V Finkelstein, S French et al. (eds) Disabling Barriers – Enabling Environments. Milton Keynes: Sage.

Oliver M (1996) Understanding Disability: From Theory to Practice. Basingstoke: Macmillan.

Oliver M (1999) The disability movement and the professions. British Journal of Therapy and Rehabilitation 6(8): 377–9.

Oliver M (2004) The social model in action. In J Swain, S French, C Barnes et al. (eds), Disabling Barriers – Enabling Environments. London: Sage.

Oliver M, Barnes C (1996) Disabled People and Social Policy. London: Longman.

Oliver M, Barnes C (1998) Disabled People and Social Policy: From Exclusion to Inclusion. Harlow: Longman.

Oliver M, Sapey B (1999) Social Work with Disabled People (2nd edn.). Basingstoke: Macmillan.

Peace S (2003) Places for care. Block 2, Unit 6 of the Open University Course. Understanding Health and Social Care (K100) (3rd edn.). Milton Keynes: Open University Press.

Pearce J, Cassar S (1999) Assessing risks. In R Steed, L Aitchison (eds), Safer Handling of People in the Community. Teddington: National Back Pain Association.

Pengelly S (1997) The Diverse and Potentially Conflicting Interpretations of Quality within Social Services. (Unpublished MBA. University of Wales Institute, Cardiff.)

Pheasant S (1986) Bodyspace: Anthropometry, Ergonomics and Design. London: Taylor & Francis.

Pheasant S (1991) Ergonomics, Work and Health. London: Macmillan.

Pheasant S (1996) Bodyspace: Anthropometry, Ergonomics and the Design of Work (2nd edn.). London: Taylor & Francis.

Pheasant S, Stubbs D (1994) Manual Handling: An Ergonomic Approach (2nd edn.). Teddington: National Back Pain Association.

Picking C (2000) Working in partnership with disabled people: New perspectives for professionals within the social model of disability. In J Cooper (ed.), Law, Rights and Disability. London: Jessica Kingsley Publishers.

Picking C, Pain H (2003) Home adaptations: User perspectives on the role of professionals. British Journal of Occupational Therapy 66(1): 2–8.

Plant R (1991) Modern Political Thought. Oxford: Blackwell.

Porteous D, Smith S (2001) Domicide: The Global Destruction of Home. Montreal and Kingston: McGill-Queens University Press.

Priestley M (1999) Disability Politics and Community Care. London: Jessica Kingsley Publishers.

Pryke M (1998) Thinking social policy into social housing. In G Hughes, G Lewis (eds), Unsettling Welfare: The Reconstruction of Social Policy. London: Routledge.

Rabiee P, Priestley M, Knowles J (2001) Whatever Next: Young Disabled People Leaving Care. Leeds: First Key.

Read J, Clements L (2001) Disabled Children and the Law: Research and Good Practice. London: Jessica Kingsley Publishers.

Reed KL, Sanderson SN (1992) Concepts of Occupational Therapy (3rd edn.). Baltimore: Williams & Wilkins.

Rees L, Lewis C (2003) Housing Sight: A Guide to Building Accessible Homes for People with Sight Problems. Cardiff: RNIB Cymru/The Welsh Assembly/JMU Access Partnership.

Rees L, Lewis C (2004) Adapting Homes: A Guide to Adapting Existing Homes for People with Sight Loss. RNIB Cymru/JMU Access Partnership.

RNIB (2002) Changing the Way We Think about Blindness: Myth and Reality. London: RNIB.

Robertson L (1996) Clinical reasoning, Part 1: The nature of problem solving, a literature review. British Journal of Occupational Therapy 59(4): 178–82.

Robinson BC (1983) Validation of a caregiver strain index. Journal of Gerontology 38(3): 344–8.

Rush A (2004) Ergonomics 24/7: Work, Life, Balance. National Back Exchange Annual Conference. Bariatrics and Ergonomics (lecture notes) 20–22 September 2004.

Salmen J (2001) US Accessibility Codes and Standards: Challenges for Universal Design. In W Preiser, E Ostroff (eds), Universal Design Handbook. New York: McGraw-Hill.

Schell B (1998) Clinical reasoning: The basis for practice. In ME Neistadt, EB Crepeau (eds), Willard and Spackman's Occupational Therapy (9th edn.). Philadelphia: Lippincott.

Schell B, Cervero R (1993) Clinical reasoning in occupational therapy: An integrative review. American Journal of Occupational Therapy 47: 605–10.

Schön D (1983) The Reflective Practitioner: How Professionals Think in Action. New York: Basic Books.

Scotland (1998) Housing for Varying Needs: A Design Guide, Part 1: Houses and Flats. Edinburgh: TSO.

Scottish Office (1998) Modernising Community Care: Guidance on the Housing Contribution.

Seligman MEP (1975) Helplessness: On Depression, Development, and Death. New York: WH Freeman.

Shearer A (1981) Disability: Whose Handicap? Oxford: Blackwell.

Social Services Inspectorate Wales (2001) Performance Management: A Strategy for Social Services in Wales. Wales: Social Services Inspectorate.

Stewart B (2000) Living space: The changing meaning of home. British Journal of Occupational Therapy 63(3): 105–10.

Stewart J (2004) Housing and independent living. In J Swain, S French, C Barnes et al. (eds), Disabling Barriers – Enabling Environments (2nd edn.). London: Sage.

Stewart J, Harris J, Sapey B (1999) Disability and dependency: origins and futures of 'special needs' housing for disabled people. Disability and Society 14(1): 5–20.

Stewart S (1999) The use of standardised and non-standardised assessments in a social services setting: Implications for practice. British Journal of Occupational Therapy 62(9): 417–23.

Stewart S, Neyerlin-Beale J (2000) The impact of community paediatric occupational therapy on children with disabilities and their carers. British Journal of Occupational Therapy 63(8): 373–9.

Stone E (1999) Disability and development in the majority world. In E Stone (ed.), Disability and Development: Learning from Action and Research on Disability in the Majority World. Leeds: The Disability Press.

Storey MF (2001) Principles of Universal Design. In W Preiser, E Ostroff (eds), Universal Design Handbook. New York: McGraw-Hill.

Stubbs R, Atwal A, McKay E (2004) Evaluating the community dependency index in a social services context. International Journal of Therapy and Rehabilitation 11(6): 281–6.

Sun (2004A) 40st man trapped, 21 July, p. 27.

Sun (2004B) 216kg (34 stone) woman stuck to sofa, 24 August, p. 28.

SBC (Syniad Benchmarking Centre) (2001) Housing Adaptations for People with Disabilities Good Practice Guides. Pembrokeshire: Syniad Benchmarking Centre.

Taylor C (1999) Occupational Therapists: Empowers or Oppressors? A Study of Occupational Therapy Students' Attitudes to Disabled People. (Unpublished PhD. Dept. Sociology, University of Warwick.)

The Stationery Office (2004) Official Documents. The Prevalence of Disability. <www.official-documents.co.uk>, accessed 29/09/04.

Thomas Pocklington Trust (2003) Housing and Support Needs of Older People with Visual Impairment – Experiences and Challenges. Occasional Paper. London: Thomas Pocklington Trust.

Thorpe S (1994) Reading and Using Plans. London: Centre for Accessible Environments.

Tinnetti ME, Richman D, Powell L (1990) Falls efficacy as a measure of falling. Journal of Gerontology 45(6): 239–43.

Townsend E (1997) Enabling Occupations: An Occupational Therapist Perspective. Ottawa: CAOT Publications ACE.

United States of America (1988) Fair Housing Amendments Act (1988) Washington: US Department of Housing and Urban Development. <www.hud.gov>, accessed 20/03/05.

United States of America (1990) Americans with Disabilities Act 1990. Washington: US Department of Justice.

Walker A (1995) Universal access and the built environment – or from glacier to garden gate. In G Zarb (ed.), Removing Disabling Barriers. London: Policy Studies Institute.

Weerdmeester JD, Weerdmeester B (2001) Ergonomics For Beginners: A Quick Reference Guide (2nd edn.). London: Taylor & Francis.

Welsh Assembly Government (2000) Circular 14/2000 Local Government: Best Value – Guidance to Local Authorities in Wales on Best Value. Cardiff: National Assembly for Wales.

Welsh Office (1978) Circular 104/78. Cardiff: Welsh Office.

Welsh Office (1996) Circular 59/96. Cardiff: Welsh Office.

West Lothian Council (1998) New Housing Partnership Initiative. Opening Doors for Older People.

Wilkinson A, Willmott H (eds) (1995) Making Quality Critical. London: Routledge.

Williams G (2002a) Home Care Technology Assessment Software for West Lothian. Phase 1 Report. Technology in Healthcare Ltd.

Williams G (2002b) Home Care Technology Assessment Software for West Lothian. Phase 2 Report (Work in Progress). Technology in Healthcare Ltd.

Wilson JR (1995) A framework and a context for ergonomics methodology. In JR Wilson, EN Corlett (eds), Evaluation of Human Work (2nd edn.). London: Taylor & Francis.

Wilson JR, Corlett EN (1995) Evaluation of Human Work. London: Taylor & Francis.

Winfield J (2003) Best adaptations redeeming people's homes: Enlightened occupational therapy. British Journal of Occupational Therapy 66(8): 376–7.

WHO (World Health Organisation) (2001) International Classification of Functioning, Disability and Health. Geneva: WHO.

Index